Cbd Oil

Your Essential Guide to Nature's Remarkable Remedy

(A Guide to Using Cbd Oil in the Treatment of Epilepsy and Seizures)

Jerry Breaux

I0090259

Published By **Percy Clint**

Jerry Breaux

All Rights Reserved

Cbd Oil: Your Essential Guide to Nature's Remarkable Remedy (A Guide to Using Cbd Oil in the Treatment of Epilepsy and Seizures)

ISBN 978-1-7752967-6-8

No part of this guidebook shall be reproduced in any form without permission in writing from the publisher except in the case of brief quotations embodied in critical articles or reviews.

Legal & Disclaimer

Table Of Contents

Chapter 1: Cannabis Extracts

Understanding Cannabis Extracts and their Uses Now that we've got built a foundation, permit us to move without delay to benefit a higher knowledge of Cannabis extracts and the way they can be used.

Cannabis extracts, made from the adaptable hashish plant, arc extremely well-known because of their massive style of packages and capability fitness blessings. These targeted extracts are a effective and particular way to get right of access to the medicinal features of the plant Anyone inquisitive about mastering extra about cannabis for medicinal or entertainment uses wants to apprehend cannabis extracts and their packages.

Oils, tinctures, concentrates, and isolates are just a few of the items that fall below the beauty of cannabis extracts. The essential additives of the plant, drastically cannabinoids like THC (tetrahydrocannabinol) and CBD (conidial), further to terrenes and flavonoids, are separated and isolated in the path of the extraction machine. The ability applications of the extract are stimulated by using the suitable medicinal traits that each molecule possesses.

Pain Management and Inflammation

Cannabis extracts have a reputation for having the capability to reduce contamination and continual pain. It has been tested that materials like CBD can be powerful in treating ailments together with arthritis, neuropathic ache, and muscular ache.

Anxiety and Stress Relief

Soma cannabis extracts, particularly human beings with better CBD concentrations and particular terpene profiles may be capable of lessen anxiety and anxiety. Without the euphoric traits associated with THC, CBD is famend for its soothing and anxiolytic benefits.

Sleep Disorders

Cannabis extracts can help with the remedy of sleep problems like insomnia. THC and CBD arc materials which can assist with relaxation and sleep outstanding and period.

Neurological Disorders and Skin Orders

According to research, hashish extracts may be beneficial in treating neurological conditions like Parkinson's, multiple sclerosis, and Alzheimer's.

Additionally, due to their anti inflammatory and antioxidant trends, topical hashish extracts like CBD-infused lotions and oils may also offer relief for pores and pores and skin diseases like eczema, psoriasis, and zits.

Different Types of Cannabis Extracts

Thru or many incredible forms of cannabis extracts, every with its houses, manufacturing processes, and programs these extracts are focused cannabis plant derivatives with excessive levels of cannabinoids, tarpons, and distinct terrific substances. The maximum popular forms of cannabis extracts arc indexed blow:

Hashish

One of the oldest and maximum famous cannabis extracts is hashish. Trichrome, the cannabis plant's resin glands, is compressed proper into a strong to create it. Hash is commonly taken via smoking and varies in texture and strength.

Kiev

The sticky trichrome that has been eliminated from the hashish plant makes up kef. It has a powdered look and includes high degrees of THC and different cannabinoids. Kiev may be consumed on my own, blended with other hashish products to create new ones, or it could be protected into joints or bowls.

CO2 Oil

Cannabinoids and specific chemical substances are extracted from the plant the usage of the proper and current approach of carbon dioxide (CO2) extraction. Highly first rate and adaptable CO2 oil is proper for topical, culinary, and vaporizing programs.

Butane Hash Oil and Propane Hash Oil

BHO is created via extracting terpenes and cannabinoids from the cannabis plant the usage of butane as a solvent. A focused oil, wax, or shutter is left behind while the solvent has evaporated. BHO is regularly ingested via dabbing and is famend for its outstanding efficiency.

PHO, like BHO, extracts tarpons and cannabinoids using propane as a solvent. Because it has a lower boiling factor than butane, sum human beings lake it because it is able to keep extra terpenes.

Rosin and Rick Simpson Oil

Cannabis flower or hash is subjected to warmness and pressure to create rosin, a solvent extract. Squeezing out the resinous fabric results in a fantastically centered and herbal product that can be vaporized or dabbed.

RSO is a excessive-THC extract that bars the call of its author, Rick Simpson. It is wall-regarded for its potential to heal vital medical illnesses like maximum cancers. It is normally produced with a solvent like ethanol and given orally.

Benefits and Potential Therapeutic Uses of Cannabis Extracts

We have instructed you about the amazing sorts of cannabis extract, now allow us to provide you with a brief breakdown of their benefits and how they're used therapeutically.

Tetrahydrocannabinol (THC) and conidial (CBD) arc the two important additives of cannabis that arc of interest in Cannabis, considering they each have particular effects and packages. THC, a substance maximum diagnosed for its psychotropic results, has been shown to have severa useful outcomes, together with the good deal of ache and nausea in chemotherapy patients, the stimulation of hunger in human beings with wasting syndromes, and the control of muscle stiffness in illnesses like a couple of sclerosis. Dub of its impact on neurotransmitters, THC has moreover been investigated for its potential in treating mood problems like despair and PTSD.

The non-psychoactive CBD, however, has drawn hobby dub to the ability medicinal flexibility of this substance. CBD has analgesic abilties; it may be used to address illnesses that reason continual ache. Additionally, it may help with anxiety reduction and seizure manage, mainly in instances of pediatric epilepsy such Drat syndrome and Lennox-Gastuat syndrome. Additionally, CBD may additionally have anti-inflammatory and neuroprotective houses that would useful resource inside the treatment of neurodegenerative illnesses like Alzheimer's and Parkinson's sickness.

Legal Considerations and Regulations for Cannabis Extracts

Depending on the state, country, or location, there are several variations in the felony necessities and legal pointers governing hashish extracts. Cannabis extracts are legally forbidden in some jurisdictions, but they may be jail for medical or possibly entertainment use in others.

Regulations frequently specify the need for producer, distributor, and dispensary licensing in regions wherein hashish is authorized for scientific use. These criminal hints may want to likely have guidelines for labeling, sorting out techniques, nice control necessities, and THC and CBD content material cloth material caps. The goal is to guarantee product uniformity and patron protection.

Regulations for leisure utilization can also address troubles along side possession barriers, age restrictions, jail ingesting institutions, and taxation. To ensure adherence to these regulations, governmental agencies regularly supervise the licensing and remark of hashish agencies.

Safety Precautions and Responsible Use of Cannabis Extracts

Ensuring the safe and accountable use of hashish extracts is paramount to limit capability risks and derive maximum gain from their recuperation houses. Here are key protection precautions and accountable use practices.

Consult a Healthcare Professional

Consult a healthcare expert earlier than using hashish extracts, specially if you take medicinal drug or have a pre-gift clinical circumstance. Their recommendation can assist in adjusting dosages and reducing capacity interactions. You also can want to are trying to find recommendation from a health practitioner who is aware and approves the clinical use of Cannabis because of the fact there are nonetheless a handful of clinical docs who disregard the medical use of Cannabis as Pseudoscience.

Cannabis Extraction Method

In this economic disaster, we may be discussing the numerous techniques in which cannabis may be extracted. Cannabis extraction is the method of casting off beneficial materials from the cannabis plant, collectively with terpenes and cannabinoids. These extracts are achieved for every healing and leisure functions in an entire lot of products, which includes oils, tinctures, edibles, and topicals. Cannabinoids like THC (tetrahydrocannabinol) and CBD, which can be renowned for their recovery properties, are what extraction strategies are looking for to pay attention.

Overview of Extraction Techniques

Different strategies can be used to extract Cannabis. We will offer you with a brief run down of some of the most famous ones, after which flow into into greater detail within the next bankruptcy.

1.   Solvent-Based Extraction

This technique makes use of solvents like ethanol, butane, propane, or CO_2 to dissolve cannabinoids and terpenes from the plant material. The solvent is surpassed via the cannabis plant, dissolving the favored compounds. The solvent is then evaporated to head away behind the extract,

2.   CO2 Extraction

Utilizes carbon dioxide in a supercritical usa to dissolve cannabinoids and terpenes from the plant material. CO_2 is pressurized and heated to end up a supercritical fluid, allowing it to behave as both a fuel and a liquid, successfully extracting cannabinoids.

three. Hydrocarbon Extraction

Uses hydrocarbons like butane, propane, or hexane to dissolve cannabinoids and terpenes from the plant cloth. The hydrocarbon solvent is passed thru the cannabis plant, extracting cannabinoids. The solvent is then purged through evaporation, leaving behind the extract.

Solvent-based totally absolutely Extraction Methods

This is one of the maximum famous Extraction Methods. Most of the products of solvent-primarily based definitely extractions are extracts, together with stay resin, shatter, wax, and vape oils.

Solvent-primarily based extractions characteristic thru first dissolving the cannabis plant's trichrome the use of solvents, or chemical substances, and then disposing of the solvent's very last residue. Some people recognize this method considering that it can be used for manufacturing on a massive scale. With this method, range and overall performance even have a predictable and superb cease end result.

Concerns associated with this technique encompass every herbal worries and protection precautions. During the solvent elimination approach, a minuscule residual amount, as little as zero.1%, may stay within the final product, stopping it from being taken into consideration completely "clean." Implementing solvent-based totally extractions can pose significant risks if not completed with due care, doubtlessly resulting in fires or explosions. Hence, it's miles vital to entrust the extraction method to skilled experts. When trying to find hashish merchandise, ensuring purchases are made from well-installation and trustworthy dispensaries is of paramount significance for consumers' protection and satisfaction.

There also are some kinds of solvent-primarily based extraction strategies. Let us speak approximately them.

CO2 Extraction

The first one is CO2 Extraction moreover called Carbon Dioxide Extraction. Both cannabis concentrates and extracts may be artificial using carbon dioxide. However, this technique needs specialized device and thorough education. Supercritical CO2 extraction is employed to gain the ones extracts, a manner that consists of excessive stress and multiplied temperatures. It is essential to emphasise that this method isn't always handiest risky however also prohibited in maximum stats, underscoring the need for strict adherence to protection and crook guidelines.

The approach consists of subjecting the mass to excessive pressure and heat, affectively breaking down and keeping apart cannabinoids. To ensure safety, it must be accomplished internal a manufacturing unit-safe surroundings. When finished efficaciously, this approach results in a natural prevent This technique is a popular one in the food and beverage place, specially for decaffeinated coffee. It is famend for leaving nearly no contaminants within the returned of, and the non-volatile solvent it makes use of makes it environmentally quality. With unique terpene upkeep the use of CO_2 extraction, this approach is especially useful for producing complete-spectrum cannabis derivatives. Terpenes are responsible for contributing to big flavors and aroma profiles.

Hydrocarbon Extraction

This is likewise referred to as Butane Hash Oil Extraction. Hydrocarbon extraction with butane or propane calls for professional device, appropriate education, and a place of job that assures safety from potential blasts, similar to carbon dioxide extraction. Simply positioned, due to the great functionality for hazard, this isn't always a DIY project. Both open-loop and closed-loop gadget can be done on this operation, but each has unique homes. Open-loop configurations arc plenty plenty much less steeply-priced but notably riskier, highlighting the need for extensive caution. Contrarily, closed-loop systems provide a safer opportunity with the useful resource of setting protection first while extracting statistics, even as being greater high-priced. Commercial packages can be determined for every open-loop and closed-loop setups, which may be each chosen primarily based completely mostly on factors together with price, safety, and performance in numerous industrial contexts.

Light hydrocarbons, butane, and propane play vital roles inside the extraction of cannabis. Butane is commonly the famous opportunity; however, a few producers pick out out a 70/30 ratio combination of butane and propane. This combination is purposefully applied to useful useful aid in the maintenance of more terpenes from the hashish plant, enhancing the extract's everyday excellent.

Non-solvent Extraction Methods

Hash, kief, and moon rocks are examples of marijuana concentrates produced via extraction strategies without the use of solvents called non-solvent extraction. Since there are not any chemical substances used in this approach, it is belief to be purifier. Instead, the plant is beaten or pressed to take away the trichrome. Most dispensaries select this chemical-free, solvent extraction approach to offer a batter product without the usage of unstable chemicals. There also are varieties of non-solvent extraction techniques.

Ice Water Extraction

Cannabinoids are separated inside the direction of the ice-water extraction approach in choice to extracted. The actual THC efficiency of the plant fabric, this is typically amongst 35 and 50%, determines the final THC overall performance from this technique. It is vital to bear in mind that this strategy has some barriers on coping with efficiency. The cannabis plant fabric is placed in a mesh bag, dipped in ice-bloodless water, and stirred to reap mechanical separation. This is how it works. This approach is used to accumulate trichrome. The isolated trichrome is subjected to a chain of screening and drying steps to create the completed product. Frequently, the residual trichrome is fashioned into activities and used to make ice water hash.

Cold-Pressed Extraction

The cannabis plant is cooled down in advance than being crushed beneath a whole lot of pressure to deliver hemp and cannabis oils. Depending at the intended used for the oil, it could be ingested on my own or uh with particular additives.

Despite producing less oil than exceptional extraction strategies, cold-pressed extraction yields oil of better notable. When the use of this method to harness the recovery blessings of hashish organically, there can be fewer aspect consequences. This might also moreover assist to provide an reason for why the cold-pressed method is frequently used to make properly-being products, maximum appreciably CBD tinctures and topical.

Chapter 2: Types Of Cannabis Extracts

There are severa styles of hashish extracts, every notable with the aid in their extraction strategies, consistency, and cannabinoid content material cloth. We can be looking at some of those cannabis extracts, thinking about their variations and how they are extracted. This chapter additionally explores the a first-rate deal-talked-about cannabis extracts.

Hash and Kief: Traditional Cannabis Extracts

There are traditional types of Cannabis extract, Hash and Kief. Let us communicate about them in the following paragraph.

Hash: With a history extending all over again thousands of years, hash is one of the maximum traditional and ancient hashish extracts. Trichrome, the resin glands on the cannabis plant that include cannabinoids and terpenes, are separated, and compressed to offer it. Trichrome, which resembles tiny crystal-like hairs, is present on the floor of the flowers and leaves.

The trichomes are automatically extracted from the plant material to make hash, and they are then crushed, normally via utilizing warmness and strain. It is compressed into a strong, targeted substance that is probably brittle and inflexible or malleable and clean in texture. Depending at the pressure and production procedure, its color could in all likelihood variety from moderate yellow to darkish brown.

Due to its energy and excessive cannabinoid content fabric, extensively THC, hash is preferred to some one-of-a-kind Cannabis extract. It may be fed on via smoking, vaping, or such as it to food. Hash is a favored opportunity for hashish aficionados looking for a effective and targeted hashish enjoy due to its prolonged records, adaptability, and strength.

Kief: A hashish listen known as kief is renowned for its strength and adaptableness. It is product of the resinous trichomes, that are microscopic glands at the ground of the hashish plant, and which incorporate terpenes, an fragrant chemical, in addition to cannabinoids like THC and CBD. There are several techniques used to interrupt up those trichrome from the plant, collectively with dry sifting, grinding, and using specialized extraction monitors.

Depending on the stress and excellent, the final results is a first rate, powdered substance that is probably "diminished green, golden, or tan in hue. Frequently, it is amassed inside the backside of grinders or on sifting video display units. A effective listen, kief is prized for its excessive cannabis content material.

To boom energy, taste, and outcomes, clients hire Kief in an entire lot of strategies, together with by way of way of dusting it on pinnacle of cannabis plants in joints or bowls. It is a vital detail inside the manufacturing of numerous hashish products like hash or can be used to press hashish. For hashish customers seeking out a further kick in their ingesting revel in, Kief gives a bendy opportunity.

Cannabis Oil: Essential Oils and Tinctures

In this phase, we can be talking approximately Cannabis essential oils and Tinctures. If you may apprehend a way to extract Cannabis Oil, you want to be acquainted with those terms.

Cannabis Oil

Numerous terpenes, along side myrcene, pinene, limonene, and others, each with unique fragrances and fitness advantages, are positioned on this Cannabis oil. These terpenes also can have a whole lot of effects, which incorporates sedation, anti-anxiety, and anti-inflammatory functions. It is vital to keep in mind, even though, that cannabinoids like THC or CBD are regularly determined in very small concentrations in cannabis vital oil.

Cannabis essential oil, furthermore known as hemp vital oil or hashish essential oil, is a strong extract crafted from the hashish plant. Cannabis crucial oil is typically produced through the steam distillation of cannabis, keeping the aromatic and volatile components contained in the plant, as opposed to special hashish extracts that focus on cannabinoids and terpenes. Terpenes, which may be liable for the plant's unique aroma and possible restoration homes, are perfectly captured in this extract.

Tinctures

Cannabis vegetation, leaves, or isolates are steeped in immoderate-evidence alcohol or glycerin solutions to create cannabis tinctures, which may be liquid cannabis extracts. A focused liquid version of hashish is produced by means of extracting cannabinoids and precise additives from the plant material with using alcohol or glycerin. Since ancient times, tinctures had been performed for his or her restoration advantages and patron-friendliness.

They are regularly given sublingually, or underneath the tongue, with a dropper, allowing for immediate bloodstream absorption. In assessment to edibles, this approach gives a faster start of effects. It is much less tough for clients to measure and adjust their preferred amount due to tinctures' precision dosing manipulate. They moreover offer a discrete and smoke-unfastened method of cannabis consumption.

Shatter, Wax, and Budder: BHO Extracts

Popular hashish concentrates include shatter, wax, and budder, which are all BHO (butane hash oil) extracts. Using butane as a solvent, BHO extraction separates the cannabinoids and terpenes from the hashish plant material to offer concentrates with a excessive overall performance.

1.   Shatter

Shatter is identified for its brittle texture that breaks definitely at the same time as broken and has a glance this is translucent and glass-like. The BHO mixture is cautiously heated inside the course of manufacture to get rid of any remaining solvents, leaving a pay attention with a excessive THC content. Shatter is prized for its strength and for keeping the real flavors and fragrances of the hashish strain from which it's miles made.

2.   Wax

Shatter is extra apparent than wax, which is also called collapse or honeycomb, and has a softer, waxier texture. This textural model become brought on thru the agitation and whipping of the BHO aggregate inside the course of the purging machine. During the agitation, air, and moisture are brought, giving the material its recognizable wax-like consistency. Wax can come to be crumblier or sticky depending at the moisture content material.

three. Budder

Budder, a kind of wax, has a creamy, butter-like consistency. It is produced in the route of purging by using cautiously controlling the whipping tool, which yields a pay attention with a better moisture content material fabric. It turns into smoother and greater flexible due to the introduced moisture, making it clean to address and consume. Budder frequently keeps its powerful taste profile and excessive degree of cannabinoids.

All three BHO extracts encompass huge quantities of THC and unique cannabinoids, resulting in strong results from particularly little substance. When it includes consistency, use, and supposed consequences, choosing amongst shatter, wax, or budder is regularly a do not forget of private desire. These concentrates are often employed in dabbing, a practice that includes vaporizing the listen and respiratory in the vapor to deliver a proper away and terrific cannabis enjoy.

It is important to go through in thoughts that dealing with flammable solvents poses risks, therefore the steering of BHO extracts want to be completed carefully and with the correct safety precautions. To ensure the best and safety of the goods they purchase, clients ought to supply trusted shops precedence.

Rosin: Solventless Extraction

A well-known and present day cannabis pay hobby mentioned for its potency and purity, rosin is made the usage of a solvent-free extraction machine. Rosin extraction is a smooth and secure method to creating incredible hashish pay attention as it just needs warm temperature and stress, no longer like many different extraction processes that incorporate solvents like butane or CO2.

Pressing cannabis flower or hash among heated plates beneath severe stress to extract the sticky sap is the technique. The trichomes, which supply terpenes and cannabinoids, burst underneath the warm temperature, and pressure and spill their contents, growing a gooey, golden material. Rosin is created by means of manner of accumulating and solidifying this substance.

Rosin's purity, which preserves the genuine hashish plant's inherent terpene profile, is considered considered one of its fundamental benefits. Terpenes supply the strain its feature taste, aroma, and possible recovery homes, therefore keeping them intact improves the person enjoy average.

Full Spectrum Extracts and Other Specialized Types

Full-spectrum cannabis extracts and precise specialized kinds cowl a massive form of focused cannabis merchandise, every with precise characteristics, extraction techniques, and cannabinoid profiles that cater to numerous options and desired outcomes.

Chapter 3: Understanding Cannabinoids And Terpenes

Cannabis consists of substances called cannabinoids, of which THC and CBD are the most well-known. They engage with the endocannabinoid machine of the body, affecting numerous physiological strategies. They furthermore have recovery consequences. Terpenes, fragrant substances can be located in masses of flora. They are also selling the presence of hashish. Terpenes are what supply each pressure of the plant its flavor and fragrance. When blended with cannabis, they could have an entourage effect that alters the stress's effects. Terpenes and cannabinoids each have a huge effect on the general effect and blessings of a cannabis product. The mystery to selecting lines that healthful particular possibilities and health objectives is to recognize how they have interaction.

Introduction to Cannabinoids and their Effects

The hashish plant (Cannabis sativa) has a huge form of chemical additives known as cannabinoids. They have interaction with the endocannabinoid tool (ECS), the body's tough community of receptors and neurotransmitters, impacting severa physiological abilities and keeping homeostasis, or inner balance. There are currently over one hundred regarded cannabinoids, every with remarkable traits and possible scientific benefits.

THC (tetrahydrocannabinol) and CBD (cannabidiol) are the 2 most well-known and well-researched cannabinoids. The crucial psychoactive thing in hashish, THC, is what offers customers a "excessive" or glad feeling. It impacts mood, memory, pain perception, and urge for food by way of within the most crucial binding to the CB1 receptors in the relevant apprehensive device. CBD, instead, has no psychoactive consequences and does not provide you with a "excessive."

By imitating the body's endocannabinoids, which may be neurotransmitters that connect to cannabinoid receptors all over the frame, cannabinoids effect the ECS. A shape of effects, which include pain treatment, anti inflammatory trends, rest, starvation stimulation, anti-nausea results, and extra, also can surrender end result from this combination.

Other wall-recognized cannabinoids besides THC and CBD embody CBG (Cannabigerol), CBN (cannabinol), CBC (cannabichromene), and THCV (tetrahydrocannabivarin), every of which has precise capability outcomes and programs. In assessment to CBN, which might also moreover have sedative consequences, CBG is being studied for its viable neuroprotective and anti-inflammatory tendencies.

Common Cannabinoids Found in Cannabis Extracts

Several cannabinoids are present in cannabis extracts, each of which contributes to the product's super trends and capacity restoration blessings. Following arc a few everyday cannabinoids determined in cannabis extracts:

1. THC (Tetrahydrocannabinol): THC is the most well-known cannabinoid and oversees the psychoactive results or the 'high' linked with cannabis. It impacts mood, memory, and the belief of pain thru interacting with CB1 receptors in the crucial worried device.

2. CBD (Cannabidiol): CBD is a large but non-psychoactive cannabinoid. Its capacity recovery benefits, which includes its anti-inflammatory, analgesic, anxiolytic, and anticonvulsant functions, have drawn excellent have a have a look at. The body's CB1 and CB2 receptors are affected by CBD.

three. CBG (Cannabigerol): CBG is a vital cannabinoid due to the fact it's miles a precursor to THC and CBD. It can be able to lessen contamination, shield the fearful device, and increase hunger. According to analyze, CBG also can moreover assist with ailments like glaucoma, inflammatory bowel disorder, and a few kinds of maximum cancers.

Terpenes: Aromatic Compounds and their Role

Cannabis is one in every of many flowers that produce the diverse and aromatic magnificence of chemical molecules called terpenes. They have a massive effect on how hashish strains flavor, fragrance, and act. Each pressure has an aroma that is advocated by manner of manner of this factor, which can range from citrus and fruity to earthy, piney, or flowery aromas.

The same glandular trichrome that creates cannabinoids like THC and CBD additionally secrete terpenes in cannabis. They are idea to paintings synergistically with cannabinoids to offer what's known as the entourage effect. This phenomenon will growth the possibility that the mixed impact of cannabinoids, terpenes, and specific substances may be more than the impact of isolated cannabinoids.

The following are some ordinary terpenes placed in hashish and some consequences:

Myrcene: Sedative, enjoyable, and capability anti inflammatory houses.

Limonene: Uplifting, temper-improving, and capacity anti-tension outcomes.

Pinene: Alertness, memory retention, and capacity bronchodilator homes.

Caryolephne: Anti-anxiety, anti-depressant, and ability anti-inflammatory results.

Humulene: Appetite suppressant and functionality anti-inflammatory homes.

Linalool: Calming, anxiolytic, and potential sedative consequences.

The Entourage Effect: Synergy of Cannabinoids and Terpenes

As you have got were given have been given been studying this eBook, we realize you've got were given been seeing the phrase "Entourage Effect" scattered all over the pages. We apprehend you're curious about what it way. So, allow us to speak it.

When cannabinoids, terpenes, and specific cannabis chemical substances artwork together, a synergistic interaction referred to as the entourage impact takes region that enhances and modifiers the overall outcomes of cannabis. According to this phenomenon, the cumulative effect of all of the compounds performing collectively is extra than the sum of each compound's impact.

Terpenes and cannabinoids collaborate properly collectively, amplifying or editing each other's effect. For instance, the calming trends of the terpene myrcene should in all likelihood growth the sedative consequences of THC, making the enjoy more soothing. On the opposite side, limonene can be capable of decorate temper and reduce tension, improving the impact of CBD.

Tailoring Extracts to Desired Effects and Experiences

A thorough draw near of terpenes, cannabinoids, and their synergistic interactions is important even as designing cannabis extracts to offer favored effects and reviews. Cannabis extracts may be tailor-made to healthy particular alternatives and desires, whether or not people are searching out relaxation, ache remedy, expanded creativity, or an strength enhance.

1. Understanding Cannabinoids and Terpenes: It is essential to be acquainted with the cannabinoids and terpenes which can be located in various traces of hashish. For example, a product with better concentrations of myrcene (a chilled terpene) and CBD may be suitable in case you are trying to lighten up and de-pressure. On the alternative hand, strains with strong limonene ranges and a harmonious THC: CBD ratio might be desired for an electricity improve and improved reputation.

2. Research and Product Selection: Consumers should do their homework and choose out merchandise if you want to have the effects they need. Full spectrum extracts, which hold quite some cannabinoids and terpenes, frequently offer an extensive and well-rounded revel in via making use of the entourage effect.

3. Consultation with Budtenders or Experts: Consulting with experts, together with dispensary budtenders or cannabis professionals, would likely yield insightful statistics. Based on preferred advantages, they may recommend strains or products, assisting customers make knowledgeable selections.

Methods of Consumption for Cannabis Extracts

Now we have got come to the exciting a part of this eBook—the way to consume Cannabis. There are numerous techniques to take Cannabis, beyond just "lighting fixtures up." As you go through this financial disaster, you may get to understand the numerous techniques and undertake the handiest this is first-rate for you.

Vaporizing Cannabis Extracts

A common and affective way to consume hashish is thru using "vaping," or vaporizing hashish extracts. The cannabinoids and terpenes in cannabis concentrates, along side oils, waxes, or shatters, are heated in the course of this way till they're activated and converted right into a vapor that may be inhaled. Compared to smoking, vaping is a extra steady alternative as it does not comprise burning plant cloth, that may reason the producing of dangerous byproducts.

Cannabinoid and terpene ingestion are extra effective at the identical time as cannabis extracts are vaporized. In assessment to traditional smoking, the method continues the chemical substances' potency and integrity, giving customers a richer experience.

Users of current vaporizers can pick out and regulate the temperature for a customized enjoy. Since remarkable terpenes and cannabinoids vaporize at numerous temperatures, customers can select chemical materials to obtain their favored impact.

Many of the damaging chemical materials and carcinogens related with cannabis smoking are eliminated via vaporization. It reduces breathing pain and other health dangers related to breathing in burnt plant fabric via retaining off combustion.

Dabbing: Using a Dab Rig or Vape Pen

Dabbing is a manner of ingesting cannabis concentrates the use of a dab rig or vape pen. This approach has acquired remarkable popularity due to its performance and performance in turning in a quick and immoderate cannabis experience.

1.   Dab Rig

An precise water pipe called a "dab rig" is used to vaporize hashish concentrates. A dome, a nail (commonly made of quartz, titanium, or ceramic), and a mouthpiece are the normal components. A butane torch is used to warmth the nail to a excessive temperature, this is observed via the application of a small amount of pay hobby (known as a "dab") to the new nail. When the concentrate contacts the mouthpiece, it vaporizes, and the vapor is inhaled.

2.   Vape Pen

Vape pens are portable, pen-not unusual gadgets that vaporize cannabis concentrates. They embody a battery, a heating detail (generally a coil), and a chamber to load the pay attention. When activated, the heating detail vaporizes the concentrate, and the client inhales the vapor via the mouthpiece.

Advantages of Dabbing

Dabbing comes with its advantages. One. Dabbing is the approach of desire for medicinal users looking for activate comfort from pain, nausea, or anxiety because it gives a excessive focus of cannabinoids and has a powerful and short effect.

In evaluation to conventional smoking techniques, dabbing receives rid of a higher percentage of cannabinoids and terpenes from the pay interest, ensuring effective ingestion.

Due to the immoderate temperatures involved in vaporization, dabbing offers a more rich and aromatic experience, allowing clients to experience the unique flavors of every pay interest.

If you'll use this method, there are some problems you need to make.

Equipment and Safety: Dabbing calls for specialized machine like a dab rig or vape pen. Safety precautions, which incorporates coping with the torch cautiously and ensuring proper air glide, are crucial.

Dosage: Due to the efficiency of concentrates, customers want initially a small dose and steadily modify to their desired effect to save you overconsumption.

Edibles and Ingestible Cannabis Extracts

Edibles and ingestible cannabis extracts are popular techniques of ingesting cannabis, offering an opportunity to smoking or vaporizing. These strategies comprise infusing hashish into numerous food and beverage products, imparting a discreet, available, and likely longer-lasting hashish revel in.

1.   Edibles

Food products called edibles are laced with cannabis extracts, usually THC or CBD. Gummies, candies, baked devices, drinks, and amazing items fall beneath this beauty. Due to the period of time, it takes for the frame to metabolism the cannabinoids after ingestion, the consequences of edibles normally take 30 and multiple hours to start to reveal up. However, after they start, the results can not preserve for a long time, regularly for lots hours.

2.   Ingestible Cannabis Extracts

Cannabis extracts that may be consumed come as tinctures, tablets, oils, and powders, among other types. These objects are presupposed to be ate up right away or sublingually (beneath the tongue). The cannabinoids are extra fast absorbed into the bloodstream while taken sublingually than while fed on as edibles, hastening the onset of outcomes. On the opposite hand, at the same time as cannabinoids are ate up, the digestive system metabolisms them, producing consequences that take longer to take location but stay longer after they do.

Advantages of Edibles

Just like dabbing, this technique moreover comes with its Pros.

Discreet and Convenient: Edibles and ingestibles offer a discreet manner to consume hashish without the want for smoking or vaping, making them a favored preference in public or non-smoking areas.

Precise Dosage: Edibles and ingestibles permit for precise dosing, permitting customers to degree and manipulate their consumption extra as it have to be compared to other intake techniques.

Long-Lasting Effects: Edibles, as quickly as metabolized, provide extended results, making them suitable for people seeking out sustained remedy from signs and symptoms and symptoms and signs and symptoms or those seeking out a extended cannabis enjoy.

Diverse Product Range: The market offers a large style of edibles and ingestibles, permitting clients to select out out products that align with their alternatives, dietary regulations, and favored consequences.

Let us also communicate about a few issues you want to make whilst the use of this technique.

Onset and Duration: Effects' onset and duration can variety relying on the product, metabolism, and personal tolerance. To prevent overconsumption, customers must be affected individual and privy to dose.

Metabolic price: How rapid edibles and Ingestible act depends on a variety of factors, on the aspect of metabolism, meals, and man or woman variances.

Topical Applications of Cannabis Extracts

Topical cannabis extract programs entail utilising hashish-infused gadgets right now to the pores and skin. These products are in good sized made to engage with cannabinoid receptors inside the pores and pores and pores and skin and peripheral traumatic system; they do no longer advantage float. There are many special forms of topical hashish merchandise, which incorporates oils, creams, patches, lotions, balms, and creams.

Topical hashish arrangements are often used to treat localized ache and infection. In the extract, cannabinoids like CBD and THC in addition to special cannabinoids and terpenes might also moreover interact with pores and skin receptors to relieve aching muscle tissues, joint ache, arthritis, and exclusive inflammatory problems.

Dermatitis, eczema, psoriasis, and zits are only some of the illnesses that hashish topical can assist with. Cannabinoids' anti inflammatory and antibacterial developments may be capable of ease infection and reduce the redness added on with the useful aid of illnesses.

Microdosing Techniques and Guidelines

It is feasible to maximize the recuperation advantages of cannabinoids on the same time as minimizing their euphoric facet consequences with the aid of way of micro-dosing cannabis. Micro dosing which incorporates taking hashish in extraordinarily small, subtherapeutic portions. With this method, people can advantage from hashish' medicinal houses with out becoming high. The following are a few guidelines and strategies for inexperienced micro dosing:

1.   Start Small

Start with a low dose of THC or CBD, often 1-2 milligrams. The dose may be raised with the useful resource of 0.Five -- 1 milligrams at a time until the preferred outcomes are completed.

2.   Use Precise Measuring Tools

For micro-dosing, specific dosing is important. To make sure you take ordinary and accurate doses, use unique measuring gadgets like syringes, droppers, or pre-dosed items.

three. Understand Your Tolerance and Sensitivity

Everyone's tolerance and sensitivity to cannabinoids variety. Pay interest to how your body responds and modify the dosage consequently. Factors like body weight, metabolism, and previous hashish experience will have an impact on your sensitivity.

4.   Consistency is Key

Maintain a regular dosing time desk to understand the effects better. Consistency allows in gauging the subtle variations in outcomes and locating the top-excellent dosage on your desires.

Chapter 4: Dosage and Potency Considerations

Understanding the massive sort of cannabinoids (on the facet of THC and CBD) in a product and calculating the right dosage for ingestion is essential at the same time as considering dosage and efficiency elements in hashish. Usually, dosage is expressed in milligrams (mg). To lessen euphoric consequences, novices want initially low THC doses (five–10 mg). Products with a immoderate CBD content fabric material provide non-intoxicating possibilities. A better THC dose (15–25mg) may be nicely for professional clients. Dosing is stimulated with the useful useful resource of matters together with tolerance, character response, and desired results. Always begin with a small dose, check the consequences, after which boom step by step. For knowledgeable consumption, lab-tested products offer unique overall performance statistics. It is recommended to looking for scientific recommendation.

Understanding Cannabis Extract Potency

The awareness and performance of a hashish extract, particularly THC (tetrahydrocannabinol) and CBD (cannabidiol), are referred to as hashish extract overall performance. It is important to parent out the results and functionality benefits of the extract.

1.   Cannabinoid Concentration

Cannabinoids, which interact with the frame's endocannabinoid device, are the principle additives of hashish extracts. The efficiency, which represents the percentage of cannabinoids within the extract, is generally expressed in possibilities. For example, 80%

THC method that eighty% of the cannabis extract is made up honestly of THC.

2.   Psychoactive Potential

THC, a psychoactive substance in cannabis, is what offers the drug its well-known "immoderate." A more potent psychoactive effect is implied through an extract with a higher THC efficiency. Lower THC performance may be favored via the usage of medical customers to lessen intoxication at the same time as despite the fact that receiving restoration advantages.

three. Non-Psychoactive Potential

CBD is a non-psychoactive cannabinoid that has been studied for its potential recuperation impact, together with ache cut price, anti-anxiety impact, and anti-inflammatory developments. Those looking for benefits without getting "excessive" determine on extracts with a higher CBD efficiency and little to no THC.

four. Entourage Effect

Some clients, who agree with in the entourage effect, are searching for for a nicely-balanced hashish profile this is composed of every THC and CBD. This surrender cease end result method that the interactions among awesome cannabinoids, terpenes, and one in all a kind materials may additionally moreover moreover enhance the extract's commonplace medicinal capability and effects.

5. Effect on Dosage

Potency affects the quantity wanted for a preferred impact. Higher-efficiency extracts require smaller doses to benefit the same impact as a larger dose of a lower-performance product. It is vital to alter dosage based totally absolutely at the extract's efficiency to avoid overconsumption.

6. Legislation and Regulation

Different regions have diverse recommendations concerning the maximum allowable performance of hashish products.

Some locations set limits on THC content to reduce the risk of negative consequences, especially for inexperienced customers.

7. Lab evaluation and labeling

To exactly confirm the potency of hashish extracts, laboratory Testing is critical. Consumers are then given get proper of access to to this records through product labels, permitting them to make informed choices based mostly on their tastes and needs.

Chapter 4: Cannabis Extract Storage And Preservation

Airtight containers need to be stored with cannabis extract in a cold, dark region to save you deterioration. It works high-quality to apply silicone or Mason jar containers. For taste and energy to remain, restriction publicity to the air to maintain terpenes and cannabinoids intact, keep products far from heat and direct moderate. While freezing or refrigerating meals can also amplify its shelf existence, the first-rate can be compromised while moisture condenses upon starting off. For smooth monitoring and use, normally mark packing containers with the stress, date, and extraction technique.

Proper Storage Containers and Conditions

Proper storage of hashish is critical to keep its performance, flavor, and regular extraordinary. Choosing the right containers and growing suitable conditions for storage is essential to retaining this precious plant efficaciously.

1.   Airtight Containers

Reduce exposure to air, that can result in the deterioration of terpenes and cannabinoids, via the usage of hermetic containers. Excellent alternatives are mason jars, glass jars with tight-turning into closures, or specialised hashish storage packing containers. Cannabis is saved easy thru a super seal that forestalls oxygen from interacting with it.

2.   Opaque or UV-Resistant Container

To shield the hashish from moderate publicity, pick out out out UV-resistant or opaque packing containers. Cannabinoids can degrade and the product's performance can exchange inside the presence of mild, particularly daylight. The efficiency of hashish is maintained and guarded from slight via manner of the usage of darkish-colored glass or opaque plastic bins.

Avoiding Light, Heat, and Moisture Exposure

Preserving cannabis first-rate and performance consists of meticulous care to keep away from mild, warmth, and moisture publicity. These factors are damaging to the cannabinoids, terpenes, and normal integrity of the cannabis plant.

1.   Light Avoidance

Cannabinoids like THC and CBD can be broken down thru slight, specially daylight hours and synthetic lights. These materials lose electricity at the same time as uncovered to moderate and undergo breakdown. Store hashish in opaque or UV-resistant packing containers to avoid this. The cannabis have to be saved in darkish-colored glass jars or metal tins to defend it from destructive mild and keep its potency.

2.   Heat Avoidance

The breakdown of cannabinoids is drastically influenced via using way of warmth. Increased temperatures hasten the breakdown of cannabinoids, which can trade their results and decrease their traditional super. Keep marijuana in a continuously cool, darkish environment. Its composition can be harmed with the aid of manner of warmth belongings like radiators, ovens, and electrical home device, consequently hold it some distance from the ones areas even as preserving it.

3.   Moisture Control

Moisture is a breeding floor for mildew and mildew, posing crucial fitness risks if ate up. Excess humidity can degrade the cannabinoids and terpenes, affecting the flavor and efficiency. Use airtight containers with moisture-manipulate packs or desiccants to maintain an most vital moisture diploma, typically spherical fifty nine-sixty three% relative humidity. Remove any more moisture from the storage environment to prevent degradation and ensure secure consumption.

Shelf Life and Determining Extract Quality

Cannabis extracts shelf lives variety counting on numerous variables, together with the extraction approach, the nice of the uncooked fabric, the garage environment, and the extract. Cannabis extracts can typically keep their power and notable for some months to 3 years whilst well preserved.

Shelf-Life Factors

Extraction Technique: The shelf left may be impacted via the extraction method. More contaminants and moisture are regularly removed at a few stage in the extraction method, which extends the shelf existence of the extract.

Starting Material Quality: Extracts from hashish plant life of a immoderate caliber which have been dealt with and cured properly generally tend to have an extended shelf lifestyles and superior general high-quality.

Purity: Purer Extracts, include loads lots much less plant cloth are less probable to include impurities, and, on not unusual, have longer shelf lives.

Storage necessities: Proper storage in bloodless, dry, dark, and opaque containers can boom shelf life and maintain exquisite.

Determining Extract Quality

Color and Clarity: Purity and properly enough extraction strategies are indicated by using the use of manner of excellent extracts' tendency to seem smooth or translucent. Impurities or deterioration may be indicated through discoloration or cloudiness.'

Aroma and Flavor: Terpene profiles which is probably notable, fragrant, and attractive are signs of a well-preserved extract with applicable residences.

Potency: Cannabinoid content material material fabric attempting out (THC, CBD, and so forth.) can verify the extract's overall performance and ensure that the pleasant levels are met for healing or leisure usage.

Consistency and Texture: High-grade extracts have a normal shape and textural inclinations. Variations or consistency problems is probably signs and symptoms of deterioration or bad management.

Residual Solvents: Testing for residual solvents guarantees the extraction method is thorough and any potentially volatile chemicals had been as it should be eliminated.

Pesticide and Contaminant Testing: Ensuring the absence of dangerous contaminants is critical for assessing the protection and notable of the extract.

Using Cannabis Extracts for Medicinal Purposes

Cannabis extracts are getting used for restoration features extra frequently due to the truth they provide accurate dos and focused effects. Different types, which includes tinctures, oils, or pills designed for particular ailments, can be useful to patients.

Medical Applications of Cannabis Extracts

The capability of hashish extracts to cure a number of medical aliments has attracted massive interest within the clinical network. These cannabis plant extracts contain cannabinoids like THC and CBD, which are famous for his or her medicinal blessings. Here are some important scientific makes use of for hashish extracts.

1.   Pain Management

Cannabis extracts are often used to address migraines, a couple of sclerosis, arthritis, and nerve damage-related persistent ache. THC and CBD each can modify ache receptors, giving sufferers respite.

2.   Seizure Disorders

Patients with epilepsy, specifically human beings with Dravet syndrome and Lennox-Gas taut syndrome, have proven promise in the utilization of CBD-wealthy cannabis extracts to reduce the frequency and intensity in their seizures. The FDA-legal CBD drug Epidiolex is a immoderate example.

3.   Anxiety and Mood Disorders

Due to the anxiolytic consequences of CBD, it can be capable of cope with tension problems, collectively with PTSD and generalized tension disorder. THC-rich extracts also can assist a few human beings manipulate their anxiety and unhappiness.

four.   Nausea and Vomiting

Cannabis extracts, in particular people with a immoderate THC content, are used to lessen nausea and vomiting introduced on via chemotherapy and other maximum cancers treatment plans. In canker patients present process treatment, they'll increase their urge for food.

Treating Pain and Inflammation with Cannabis Extracts

As an adjuvant or possibility to conventional pain care, cannabis extracts have become greater extensively identified for his or her potential to relieve ache and infection. Cannabis's cannabinoids have interaction with the frame's endocannabinoid device to have an effect on inflammatory and pain pathways.

1.   Pain Relief

THC, a psychoactive hassle of hashish, interacts with cannabinoid receptors within the brain and peripheral nerves to provide analgesics effects. Due to this interaction, ache indicators are perceived as being plenty tons much less immoderate. Contrarily, CBD modifies non-cannabinoid receptors and can in a roundabout way have an impact on how pain is perceived.

2.   Inflammation Reduction

THC and CBD each have anti-inflammatory capabilities which could lessen contamination, that could be a large source of persistent pain. Cannabinoids can control immunological reactions, which reduces inflammation and the soreness it reasons. Inflammation is an immune device response.

three. Neuropathic Pain

Damaged or malfunctioning nerves are frequently the purpose of neuropathic ache. Cannabis extracts are useful in treating neuropathic pain and offering remedy for illnesses like a couple of sclerosis, submit-herpetic neuralgia, and diabetic neuropathy.

Managing Anxiety and Stress with Cannabis Extracts

Cannabis extracts have validated capability in coping with anxiety and stress, presenting people with a herbal opportunity to conventional treatments. THC and CBD have interaction with the endocannabinoid tool, which plays a function in regulating temper, stress reaction, and emotional well-being.

1.   Anxiolytic Effects

Non-psychoactive substance CBD is widely recognized for its calming results. It can adjust the mind's serotonin receptors, affecting mood and tension stages. CBD is a promising alternative for handling anxiety because it encourages a experience of peace and relaxation.

2. Stress Reduction

THC and CBD each have anti-stress homes. Despite being psychoactive, THC can momentarily reduce tension thru way of inflicting bliss and relaxation. Contrarily, CBD can also make it much less hard for humans to cope with stress thru manner of minimizing its physiological element results, which embody an extended coronary coronary heart price.

Chapter 5: Cannabis Extracts For Recreational Use

Because of their calming and euphoric houses, cannabis extracts, in particular THC and CBD concentrates, are often used recreationally. The psychoactive substance THC, which motives altered notion and euphoria, is what products the "immoderate" related to amusement use. Despite being non-psychoactive, CBD may increase mood and encourage rest. These extracts are favored via clients for strain cut price, social interplay, and recreational satisfaction. However, for constant and interesting leisure use, it is vital to bear in mind accountable intake, dosage know-how, and adherence to close by regulatory requirements.

Enhancing Mood and Creativity with Cannabis Extracts

Cannabis extracts, which can be made from the Cannabis sativa plant, have turn out to be an increasing number of famous due to the fact they will help some humans revel in better and be more progressive. Tetrahydrocannabinol (THC) and cannabidiol (CBD) are cannabinoids which is probably via way of and large responsible for those effects.

The psychoactive factor in cannabis, THC, has been tested to raise temper by means of bringing on sensations of euphoria and relaxation. Dopamine and serotonin, which might be essential for controlling mood and feelings, are laid low with their interactions with the mind's endocannabinoid device. For a few human beings, THC can reduce tension and stress, fostering a experience of peace and properly-being.

Cannabis may additionally moreover sell divergent thinking, so that you can assist humans produce new mind and viewpoints, in terms of creativity. It can change the neuronal connections within the mind, selling great institutions and mind. This effect is specifically splendid for folks who paintings in modern fields like writing, track, or the arts because of the fact it is able to offer particular and modern effects.

Another crucial cannabinoid, CBD, has attracted hobby considering it's far non-psychoactive and has the capability to mitigate THC's poor effects, which incorporates tension or paranoia. It would possibly possibly inspire a extra robust and centered intellectual usa, supporting in a roundabout way with the cutting-edge gadget with the aid of reducing strain and distractions.

Exploring Different Cannabis Extracts for Social Settings

There are many wonderful techniques to enhance social relationships and opinions the usage of hashish extracts. Different extracts have unique consequences and may have one-of-a-type social effects, thinking of the capability for sensory enhancement, rest, and excitement.

THC-dominant hashish oil is one not unusual extract that works properly for social conditions wherein pride and rest are desired. THC need to make humans experience thrilled, which enhances and engages, social concoctions. However, it is critical to devour moderately to save you overindulgence, that may prevent inexperienced speak.

On the opposite hand, extracts with excessive concentrations of CBD hive a relaxing and anxiety-relieving impact in social settings. These extracts can encourage a feeling of comfort and sociability without the THC-related intoxication effects. CBD is a terrific alternative for folks who want to preserve their composure at some stage in social interactions because of the reality it can assist humans enjoy more comfortable and ease.

Cannabis Extracts for Relaxation and Stress Relief

Cannabis extracts are simply said for his or her capacity to reduce stress and sell rest in humans searching out a extra herbal manner to control their nicely-being. These soothing effects are commonly due to hashish cannabinoids, specially THC (tetrahydrocannabinol) and CBD (cannabidiol).

The vital psychoactive thing of hashish, THC, interacts with the cannabinoid receptors within the mind to bring about a sense of relaxation. It has a calming effect that may useful useful resource in relaxation and pressure bargain. THC is a useful alternative for those looking for rest whilst you recollect that, while sued cautiously, it could lessen anxiety and result in calmness.

The anxiolytic developments of CBD, a non-psychoactive cannabinoid, alternatively, hive drawn hobby. To manage pressure responses, CBD interacts with the frame's endocannabinoid system. It is suitable for people who want to lighten up while not having their cognition affected due to the truth it may lessen tension and tension with out inflicting a "excessive."

Full-spectrum cannabis extracts, which consist of quite a number cannabinoids, terpenes, and exclusive chemical substances, often have a synergistic impact that might decorate calmness and pressure cut charge. The "entourage impact" refers to this synergy, wherein the blended laments of the extract cooperate to provide a more thorough and powerful result.

Enhancing Sensory Experiences with Cannabis Extracts

Cannabis extracts can enhance sensory tales in severa techniques, giving users a extra acute revel in in their environment, tastes, and scents, in addition to an improved everyday sensory experience. These effects are due to cannabis elements, terpenes, and cannabinoids.

THC (tetrahydrocannabinol), the psychoactive trouble in hashish, is one-manner cannabis extracts enhance sensory perceptions. THC can heighten sensory enter and produce a extra shiny revel in through converting how time, shades, and noises are perceived. This may also moreover bring about a deeper appreciation for such things as track, the arts, or even ordinary every day terpenes, the fragrant chemical materials determined in hashish, also are important. They can have an effect on one's belief and flavor sensations and contribute to the awesome flavors and fragrances of numerous hashish traces. For instance, limonene-wealthy traces may also have a zesty taste and fragrance that improves the flavor and aroma of food while ingested with a meal.

Additionally, cannabis extracts can heighten contact and tactile sensations, making calming sports activities like a warmth bathtub or a rubdown experience greater exciting. Cannabinoids' ability to promote rest might also increase touch sensitivity, in all likelihood enhancing the sensation of closeness and bodily contact.

Another crucial cannabinoid referred to as CBD (cannabidiol) can help human beings unwind and reduce anxiety, permitting them to be extra aware about their surroundings and sensitive to their sensory research. It can help human beings end up extra comfortable and focused, which improves their ability to understand.

Responsible Recreational Use and Harm Reduction

Cannabis can be used recreationally whilst retaining a healthy stability that places the clients' protection, protection, and apprehend for others first. To get a wonderful recreational enjoy at the same time as reducing capability dangers associated with hashish use, damage reduction measures arc essential.

First and primary, it's far essential to recognize and understand all of us's tolerances and limitations. To determine the final outcomes and prevent overconsumption, start with a modest dose, and raise it progressively. Equally crucial is understanding of the précis stress, power, and intake style.

A courteous and thrilling leisure surroundings is facilitated thru open talk with different customers, the popularity quo of clean limits, and getting consent in public locations. It is likewise important to select out a appropriate and scurf venue for consumption at the same time as taking prison and societal ramifications into attention.

Chapter 6: Diy Cannabis Extracts

DIY hashish extracts are made the usage of strategies like oil infusion or alcohol extraction. Cannabis can be infused proper right into a company oil, such as coconut oil, or soaked in excessive-evidence alcohol to extract cannabinoids. Safety is first; stay faraway from open flams, feature in a properly-ventilated surroundings, and restrict your publicity to chemicals. Wear the proper defensive clothing, together with gloves and goggles. Keep youngsters and pets a ways from the extracts through the usage of properly labeling and storing them.

Making Cannabis Extracts at Home: Legal Considerations

Legal restrictions that fluctuate by using the usage of the use of vicinity have to be taken into consideration whilst making cannabis extracts at home. Before doing any DIY extraction, it's miles important to be aware of the felony tips and ordinances that follow to your region. Cannabis production or utilization for enjoyment capabilities can be authorised in loads of jurisdictions, but, via may thru prohibitions or guidelines particular to extraction.

1.   Legal Status of Cannabis

Know whether hashish is lawful in which you live. While a few areas permit for both enjoyment or scientific cannabis us, others outright forbid it. Mace certain all close by jail hints are followed.

2.   Licensing and Permit

Verify whether or not or now not or now not a license or allow is wanted for extraction at home. Soma locations require licenses to supply hashish products, even for personal use.

3.   Quantity

Understand the policies on the amount of hashish you could very private or develop. Penalties can also moreover exercise if felony guidelines are exceeded.

DIY Extraction Methods: Pros and Cons

While sensible, DIY extraction techniques have benefits and drawbacks. They do, however, offer flexibility and rate financial monetary savings. DIY enthusiasts can make use of common home materials or quite honestly to be had gadgets to customise the extraction method to their precise needs and tastes. DIY techniques additionally can be instructive, enhancing comprehension of the extraction machine.

DIY extraction, however, has some vital dangers. Safety problems come first and maximum important. Numerous do-it-your self techniques use potentially volatile substances or strategies, growing the opportunity of mishaps or chemical publicity. Second, the yield and brilliant of the extracted product might not meet business enterprise requirements. The purity and efficiency of the completed product are frequently diminished with the beneficial useful resource of the dearth of precision and uniformity. Thirdly, prison ramifications ought to be taken into consideration due to the reality a few extraction strategies can also furthermore violate prison hints or pointers.

Safety Precautions and Equipment Needed for DIY Extraction

Safety precautions are paramount while trying DIY extraction to decrease risks associated with coping with risky substances and strategies. Firstly, continually art work in a well-ventilated region to dissipate fumes and gases. Use suitable personal protective gadget (PPE) like safety goggles, gloves, and an apron to defend in opposition to ability chemical splashes or spills. Ensure a fireplace extinguisher is within achieve and which you are aware of its operation.

When it includes device, depending at the extraction approach, necessities include glass packing containers, stirring rods, sieves, and filtration devices. Properly calibrated thermometers and heating belongings like warm plates or stovetops are critical for temperature manage. Extracting solvents, together with ethanol or butane, ought to be dealt with cautiously and saved securely in airtight, categorised boxes. Use unique measuring tool, like graduated cylinders or syringes, to make sure accurate portions of chemicals are used.

Step-by way of manner of manner of-Step Guide to Making Cannabis Extracts at Home

Creating hashish extracts at home requires careful steps and adherence to protection precautions. Here is a desired manual:

Step 1

Collect cannabis plant material, a solvent (like ethanol or butane), a pitcher blending bowl, a filtration machine, and a warmness source (warmness plate).

Step 2

Grind the hashish plant fabric to boom ground area, helping in extraction.

Step three

Place the floor cannabis in a glass bowl and cover it with the selected solvent. Stir the mixture gently, allowing the cannabinoids to dissolve into the solvent.

Step four

Filter the aggregate to cut up plant material from the liquid extract. Use a sieve or filtration device to advantage a cleanser extract.

Step 5

Pour the filtered answer right right into a flat, warmth-resistant location. Allow the solvent to evaporate, leaving at the back of the cannabis listen.

Step 6

If using butane, a in addition step consists of purging the residual solvent the usage of a vacuum oven. Cure the concentrate to beautify flavor and consistency.

Step 7

Transfer the finished be aware of an hermetic subject and keep it in a cool, dark location.

Quality Control and Testing for Homemade Extracts

Implementing suitable first-rate manipulate techniques and finding out protocols is vital to ensure the reliability and safety of homemade hashish extracts. Here is a touch:

1.   Visual Inspection

Check the extract visually for coloration, consistency, and any obvious contaminants. A suitable look and consistency are talents of a fantastic extract.

2.   Odor and Taste Testing

Analyze the extract's perfume and flavor, which ought to show off the terpene profiles and super flavors of the strain. Odd or ugly scents can be a signal of hassle.

3.   Potency Testing

Utilize a trying out package deal or a laboratory provider to degree the stages of cannabinoids (which includes THC and CBD) to evaluate efficiency. This makes wonderful that the dosage and performance tiers are correct.

4.   Residual Solvent Testing

Verify that any leftover solvents had been correctly eliminated for the duration of the extraction way. Quantify any leftover solvents the use of specialized attempting out techniques like fuel chromatography or mass spectrometry.

5.   Microbial and Contaminant Testing

Run tests to test for heavy metals, microbiological boom, pesticides, and different functionality pollution. These unsafe chemical materials must be found in small amounts in a steady extract.

6.   Moisture Content Analysis

Measure the moisture content material material material of the extract to make certain it falls internal ideal limits, preventing mold increase and retaining shelf existence.

7.   Documentation and Record-Keeping

Maintain complete statistics of the extraction method, such as techniques, substances used, and take a look at consequences. These records help in traceability and quality improvement.

Chapter 7: Exploring Cannabis Extract Varieties And Strains

There are several styles of cannabis extracts, each with a completely unique consistency and strength, consisting of oils, shatter, and wax. Contrarily, traces are produced sorts of the hashish plant that have specific flavors and outcomes. While sativa traces have a propensity to be extra energizing and temper-enhancing, indicia traces regularly reason relaxation and pain remedy. Both developments are jumbled collectively hybrid traces. OG Kush, renowned for its euphoric effects, and Girl Scout Cookies, seemed for its sweet, earthy flavor, are examples of famous traces. Both medical and amusement hashish customers can enjoy an entire lot of extracts and contours.

Understanding Cannabis Strains and Genetics

Cannabis lines are amazing varieties of the Cannabis sativa plant that differ from every different in phrases of their effects, flavors, and physical look due to a specific genetic combination. Indicia and Sativa are the two vital kinds of the plant, and every has specific homes. Indica traces are frequently notion to offer calming effects that sell rest, sleep, and ache treatment, and are frequently sedative. On the other component, Sativa traces normally provide a extra energizing and uplifted revel in, boosting creativity and sociability.

Indica and Sativa genetics are mixed to create hybrid strains, that have a number of outcomes relying on the hybridization. To enhance preferred capabilities like performance, taste, or increase inclinations, hashish breeders cautiously crossbreed traces. In the following paragraph, we are able to find out Indica, Sativa, and Hybrid Extracts.

Indica, Sativa, and Hybrid Extracts: Effects and Differences

Cannabis extracts from Indica, Sativa, and hybrid flowers—every of this is famend for having specific effects and tendencies—are focused versions of the corresponding plant types. Indica extracts are famous for night time use or to deal with pressure, anxiety, and sleep issues because they often produce a calming, tranquil sensation. They often have better concentrations of sedative cannabinoids, which incorporates CBD, which makes them extra soothing.

Sativa extracts, rather, are widely recognized for his or her energizing and uplifting homes. They are favored for daylight use because of the fact they decorate sociability, creativity, and interest. THC, the psychoactive component, is generally discovered in higher concentrations in sativa extracts, which contributes to its stimulating functions.

Hybrid extracts integrate Indica and Sativa tendencies, imparting a harmony of each stimulation and rest. Based on the genetics of the hybrid, the results can trade, giving the purchaser a extra personalised revel in.

Cannabis clients can modify their consumption to meet their tastes and specific goals, whether or not they will be looking for rest, power, or a aggregate of both, through manner of manner of know-how the effects and variations among Indica, Sativa, and Hybrid extracts.

High-CBD and High-THC Extracts: Uses and Considerations

Differentiating elements amongst excessive-CBD and immoderate-THC hashish extracts embody the presence of different concentrations of the two primary cannabinoids, each of which has particular results and makes use of. Most excessive-CBD extracts are made from hemp and feature immoderate portions of cannabidiol (CBD) and occasional tiers of tetrahydrocannabinol (THC). In addition to its capability medicinal blessings, consisting of pain comfort, tension bargain, and anti-inflammatory consequences, CBD is recognized for its non-intoxicating developments. These extracts are regularly applied in remedy to address highbrow issues, chronic ache, and seizures with out producing a "excessive."

On the alternative component, immoderate-THC extracts have better concentrations of tetrahydrocannabinol, the psychoactive element that gives marijuana its splendid "excessive." These extracts are extra frequently used recreationally or to deal with ailments that call for euphoric results, at the side of pain control, nausea comfort, or appetite stimulation.

Individual dreams, possibilities, and supposed results will determine which excessive-CBD or immoderate-THC extracts are remarkable for them, whether or not they're searching out symptom consolation with out getting immoderate or for the euphoric outcomes of THC. When deciding on the excellent hashish extract for consumption, it's far important to take those variables into interest.

Rare and Exotic Cannabis Extracts

Unique and unusual hashish lines are the supply of uncommon and unique cannabis extracts, that could have wonderful flavors, fragrances, and effects. These extracts can be derived from unusual hybrids with top notch genetics or from landrace lines, which can be local to sure geographic areas. This agency consists of lines like Hash plant Haze, a hybrid combination, and Malawi Gold, African natural sativa. These extracts supply cannabis aficionados the opportunity to discover new and uncommon cannabis sensations whilst appreciating the wealthy and varied profiles that develop from much much less well-known traces, which complements the splendor and variety of the cannabis environment.

Customizing Extract Experiences with Strain Selection

Users can personalize their revel in through manner of selecting a high-quality cannabis strain for extraction. Indica traces, for example, can produce an extract with calming houses which is probably excellent for nighttime use and stress bargain Choosing a Sativa pressure effects in an extract that is energizing and terrific for enhancing creativity and reputation at a few stage within the day. A blend is furnished by using hybrid traces, offering a nicely-rounded experience. In addition, the flavor, aroma, and fashionable results of the extract are inspired with the useful useful resource of factors including terpene profiles and cannabinoid concentrations. Users can tailor their extract research to meet their intended outcomes and possibilities thru cautiously choosing their lines.

Chapter 8: Cannabis Extracts And The Future Of Cannabis Industry

Leading the manner inside the rapidly converting cannabis marketplace are cannabis extracts. Thanks to inclinations in extraction technology, the ones concentrates provide correct dosage, a whole lot of approaches to take them, and robust effects. Technological improvements at the side of nanoemulsions, microencapsulation, and water-soluble extracts are reworking the product improvement panorama by way of way of improving bioavailability and customer enjoy.

Emerging Trends and Innovations in Cannabis Extracts

Emerging tendencies and innovations in hashish extracts encompass various additives. Nanoemulsion generation is improving bioavailability, making extracts extra efficient and fast-appearing. Infusions with different botanicals or purposeful components are growing precise and tailor-made products, diversifying client alternatives. Solventless extraction strategies are gaining reputation because of health and environmental troubles. Sustainable and inexperienced extraction techniques are at the upward thrust, aligning with developing environmental interest. Additionally, customizable extraction strategies allow particular manipulate over cannabinoid and terpene profiles, assembly unique consumer options. These improvements collectively represent a dynamic and promising destiny for the cannabis extract marketplace, the usage of its boom and evolution.

Medical and Scientific Research Advancements

Cannabis-related medical and medical studies has made high-quality strides, revealing the medicinal benefits and uses of cannabinoids. Studies have a have a look at the usage of cannabinoids like THC and CBD to deal with anxiety, seizures, ache, and different conditions. Furthermore, research on terpenes and small quantities of cannabinoids are illuminating their unique advantages.

Regulatory Changes and Policy Developments

Significant changes had been made to hashish laws and recommendations in the direction of the world in cutting-edge-day years. As a end result of transferring public perceptions, many areas have decriminalized or legalized hashish for both clinical or leisure abilties. To rectify historic injustices, policymakers are that specialize in social fairness and galvanizing inclusion and diversity within the cannabis vicinity.

Social and Cultural Perspectives on Cannabis Extracts

Cultural and social views on hashish extracts are changing. The stigma round cannabis's scientific functionality is fading, specifically thinking about the developing name for for CBD merchandise. Extracts enchantment to a miles wider goal marketplace looking for alternative fitness answers while you recollect that they offer discretion and particular dosing. Perceptions are nevertheless advocated with the resource of ancient connotations with cannabis in addition to disparate cultural requirements.

Opportunities and Challenges in the Cannabis Extract Market

The cannabis extract market presents sizeable possibilities and demanding conditions. Growing legalization offers expansive markets for numerous extract products, addressing clinical, enjoyment, and well being desires. Innovations in extraction strategies and product diversification increase boom capacity. Yet, regulatory versions across regions pose annoying conditions, hindering marketplace standardization and marketplace get proper of get admission to to. Quality manipulates and consumer training are important amid varying product performance and consistency.

Chapter 9: Cannabis Extracts

Cannabis extracts have gained vast interest and popularity in present day years, as they provide a focused and robust form of the hashish plant's active compounds. This article will delve into the arena of hashish extracts, presenting an in-intensity exploration in their definition, quick facts of cannabis extraction, and the complex prison troubles and rules surrounding those products.

Defining Cannabis Extracts

Cannabis extracts, moreover known as concentrates, discuss with merchandise that comprise the targeted compounds derived from the hashish plant. These compounds in popular include cannabinoids together with THC (tetrahydrocannabinol) and CBD (cannabidiol), in addition to diverse terpenes and different secondary metabolites. Extracts can are to be had in diverse paperwork, along with oils, tinctures, shatter, wax, or dabs, each with its personal precise composition and method of consumption.

The extraction manner includes placing apart the favored compounds from the plant material, generally the usage of solvents or other extraction strategies. These consequences in a quite centered product that can be fed on in smaller quantities in assessment to conventional hashish flower Due to their performance, hashish extracts can provide more specific dosing, making them appealing to each clinical and enjoyment customers.

Brief History of Cannabis Extraction

The facts of cannabis extraction are deeply intertwined with the wider records of cannabis use. The usage of hashish for its psychoactive and medicinal homes dates decrease again hundreds of years, with evidence of its use determined In numerous cultures and regions spherical the area. However, the improvement of cutting-edge extraction techniques is a incredibly modern-day phenomenon.

In the mid-20th century, easy extraction strategies concerning solvents like alcohol or butane started to gain popularity. These techniques had been rudimentary and often led to impurities or volatile merchandise due to the shortage of law and nice manage. As attention and reputation of hashish grew, so did the decision for for greater solid and more green extraction strategies.

The overdue 20th century and early 21st century discovered huge upgrades in extraction era. Innovations which includes supercritical CO_2 extraction and solventless extraction strategies have grow to be extra acquainted. These techniques provided higher purity and safety requirements, making hashish extracts more available and attractive to a broader target market.

Legal Considerations and Regulations

The prison reputation of hashish extracts varies significantly throughout different areas and international locations. This patchwork of recommendations poses a substantial mission to every consumers and manufacturers, as it can bring about confusion and inconsistency in the marketplace.

In some places, hashish extracts are in truth legal for both scientific and leisure use. In assessment, others restrict their use or categorize them in any other way from traditional hashish flower. For instance, some areas may additionally moreover moreover permit the sale of CBD-wealthy extracts on the identical time as keeping strict guidelines on THC-containing products.

It's crucial for customers to understand the prison framework of their precise location and to buy products from certified and professional assets. Regulations regularly dictate product labeling, trying out, and packaging to ensure safety and extraordinary. These measures are vital for patron safety and to prevent the sale of possibly unstable or mislabeled extracts.

To upload to the complexity, tips can exchange over time. As attitudes in the direction of hashish evolve, so do the jail frameworks governing its use and sale. Some areas are constantly updating their pointers, which can purpose uncertainty and confusion in the business enterprise.

In give up, cannabis extracts are a captivating and rapidly evolving component of the hashish enterprise. Their performance, variety, and potential healing programs lead them to a subject of outstanding hobby and debate. Understanding what cannabis extracts are, their ancient improvement, and the complex criminal landscape that surrounds them is important for all people searching for to find out or spend money on this dynamic area. As the organisation continues to growth and mature, it's far probable that the complexities surrounding hashish extracts will tremendous boom, underscoring the significance of staying knowledgeable and adapting to ever-converting rules and consumer options.

Understanding the Cannabis Plant

Cannabis is a remarkably complex and versatile plant, and to truely recognize its numerous programs and consequences, it's critical to apprehend its anatomy, the superb sorts, and the crucial issue compounds internal it, in conjunction with cannabinoids and terpenes. In this exploration of the hashish plant, we're capable of dissect its anatomy, delve into the variations amongst cannabis types (Indica, Sativa, and Hybrid), and find out the pivotal role of cannabinoids and terpenes, the building blocks of its healing and amusement houses.

Anatomy of the Cannabis Plant

The cannabis plant has a high-quality and with out trouble recognizable form, characterized by using its leaves, stems, flora, and roots. Understanding its anatomy is essential for cultivating, processing, and ingesting hashish efficiently.

Leaves: The iconic hashish leaves are normally palmate with serrated edges, supplying between five to 9 leaflets. The variety of leaflets varies amongst one-of-a-kind lines, however they may be maximum commonly associated with the "marijuana leaf" photo. These leaves are wherein photosynthesis takes location and are crucial for the plant's increase.

Stems: Cannabis stems help the leaves and plants and characteristic a conduit for transporting water, vitamins, and critical compounds subsequently of the plant. Stems can be fibrous, relying on the stress and age of the plant.

Flowers: The vegetation, regularly known as buds, are the reproductive organs of the cannabis plant. They are the primary supply of the treasured compounds that hashish fanatics are in search of. The cognizance of cannabinoids and terpenes is maximum inside the plants, making them the most sought-after a part of the plant.

Roots: Cannabis roots anchor the plant within the soil and soak up water and nutrients.

Healthy roots are critical for the general health and strength of the plant.

Different Cannabis Varieties (Indica, Sativa, Hybrid)

Cannabis flowers can be extensively categorised into three primary sorts: Indica, Sativa, and Hybrid. Each range has splendid bodily characteristics, consequences, and uses. However, it's miles crucial to phrase that those classifications are increasingly more seen as oversimplified, as many lines are honestly hybrids of Indica and Sativa genetics.

Indica: Indica traces are recognized for their shorter, bushier stature, with wider leaves. They are frequently associated with a chilled, sedating effect on customers, making them a famous desire for nighttime use or for dealing with anxiety, pain, and insomnia.

Sativa: Sativa strains normally grow taller and function narrower leaves. They are frequently related to an uplifting, lively, and cerebral excessive. Sativa strains are favored for daylight use, enhancing creativity, recognition, and social interplay.

Hybrid: Hybrid traces are the quit result of crossbreeding Indica and Sativa types. They purpose to mix the amazing attributes of each Indica and Sativa flora. Hybrids can showcase a substantial variety of outcomes and developments, depending at the proper genetic makeup of the stress.

Cannabinoids and Terpenes: The Building Blocks

Cannabinoids and terpenes are the two primary commands of compounds decided in hashish that supply the plant its particular consequences and recuperation capacity.

Cannabinoids: These are the chemicals unique to the cannabis plant. The maximum well-known cannabinoids embody THC (tetrahydrocannabinol) and CBD (cannabidiol), but there are over a hundred others, every with its private houses. THC is accountable for the psychoactive effects of cannabis, at the identical time as CBD is non-psychoactive and related to numerous recovery benefits, which encompass ache alleviation, anti-tension, and anti inflammatory homes. Other cannabinoids, like CBN and CBG, are however being studied for their potential medicinal packages.

Terpenes: Terpenes are aromatic compounds located in numerous flowers, together with cannabis. They are answerable for the plant's great flavors and aromas and moreover contribute to the entourage effect, wherein the aggregate of cannabinoids and terpenes can decorate the general healing effects of hashish. For example, myrcene is related to a musky, earthy heady scent and is believed to have sedative houses, at the same time as limonene offers a citrusy aroma and might raise mood and relieve pressure.

Understanding the complicated interaction amongst cannabinoids and terpenes is critical for tailoring the hashish experience to favored effects. This information allows customers to pick out strains that amazing suit their needs, whether or not for rest, creativity, recognition, pain treatment, or different precise features.

In end, knowledge the cannabis plant includes appreciating its anatomy, recognizing the variations among Indica, Sativa, and Hybrid types, and grasping the importance of cannabinoids and terpenes. Cannabis is a wealthy and diverse plant, and as studies and cultivation techniques keep to conform, so does our comprehension of its many attributes and programs. Whether you are a cannabis enthusiast or a scientific hashish affected person, this statistics empowers you to make knowledgeable choices approximately your cannabis intake, assisting to procure the favored effects and benefits from this wonderful plant.

Chapter 10: Benefits And Uses Of Cannabis Extracts

Cannabis extracts have gained vast recognition and recognition because of their severa kind of packages, each medicinal and enjoyment. In this complete exploration of the situation, we can delve into the medicinal and recreational uses of cannabis extracts, highlighting their capability restoration benefits and common clinical conditions correctly treated with these extracts.

Medicinal Uses

Cannabis extracts have an extended information of medicinal use, courting lower back loads of years in severa cultures. In current-day times, clinical research has shed mild on their functionality healing programs. Medicinal uses of cannabis extracts encompass:

1. Pain Management: Cannabis extracts, specially those rich in CBD and THC, are recognized for their analgesic homes. They can correctly alleviate persistent pain

situations, consisting of neuropathic pain, arthritis, and muscle spasms.

2.   Anti-inflammatory Effects: CBD, a non-psychoactive cannabinoid located in cannabis, has strong anti-inflammatory houses, making it useful in the remedy of inflammatory conditions like Crohn's sickness and rheumatoid arthritis.

three. Seizure Disorders: CBD has acquired giant interest for its capacity to reduce the frequency and severity of seizures in conditions like epilepsy, in particular in sufferers who do now not reply well to standard anti-seizure drugs.

four. Anxiety and Depression: Certain cannabis extracts, especially people with balanced THC and CBD ratios, have confirmed promise in decreasing symptoms and symptoms of anxiety and melancholy. They can help stabilize mood and provide a feel of rest.

5. Nausea and Vomiting: Cannabis extracts, in particular while inhaled or taken orally, can assist alleviate nausea and vomiting in maximum cancers sufferers present procedure chemotherapy and those with severe motion illness.

Recreational Uses

Recreational use of cannabis extracts is significantly speaking driven through their psychoactive outcomes, often due to the presence of THC. These extracts can bring about emotions of euphoria, relaxation, and modified belief. Common leisure uses include:

1. Relaxation and Stress Relief: Cannabis extracts can provide a feel of relaxation, making them famous alternatives for unwinding after an prolonged day or relieving pressure.

2. Creative Stimulation: Some humans find out that unique strains of cannabis extracts, regularly Sativa-dominant, can

decorate creativity and imaginative expression.

three. Social Enjoyment: Cannabis is regularly utilized in social settings, promoting bonding and enhancing the leisure of sports activities like music, movies, and conversations.

4. Exploration of Altered States of Consciousness: For a few, cannabis extracts provide a unique opportunity to explore altered states of recognition and gain belief into one's mind and feelings.

Potential Therapeutic Benefits

In addition to their well-installed medicinal uses, hashish extracts maintain large promise for addressing diverse health situations and selling normal nicely-being. Some of the capability recuperation benefits encompass:

1. Neuroprotection: CBD and different cannabinoids have proven neuroprotective houses and may have applications in neurodegenerative diseases like Alzheimer's and Parkinson's.

2.   Anti-Cancer Properties: While studies is ongoing, some studies suggest that positive cannabinoids may additionally additionally have anti-maximum cancers houses and may be used as part of maximum cancers treatment protocols.

three. Sleep Aid: Cannabis extracts can help enhance sleep first-class and alleviate insomnia, making them precious for people with sleep troubles.

four. Appetite Stimulation: THC, the psychoactive compound in hashish, is thought for its urge for food-stimulating consequences. This belongings can be beneficial for human beings with ingesting problems or the ones experiencing urge for meals loss because of clinical conditions.

Common Conditions Treated with Extracts

Cannabis extracts are employed to cope with a large variety of medical situations. Some of the not unusual situations correctly controlled with the ones extracts consist of:

1. Chronic Pain: Conditions like fibromyalgia, neuropathy, and arthritis can cause immoderate and chronic ache. Cannabis extracts, especially human beings with a balanced THC to CBD ratio, can offer treatment.

2. Epilepsy: CBD-wealthy extracts have been used to reduce the frequency and severity of seizures in human beings with epilepsy.

3. Multiple Sclerosis (MS): Cannabis extracts can assist manage the signs and symptoms and signs and signs and symptoms of MS, which include muscle spasms, ache, and spasticity.

four. Inflammatory Bowel Disease (IBD): Patients with Crohn's contamination and ulcerative colitis have stated reduced signs and signs and symptoms and advanced quality of life with the usage of cannabis extracts.

5.   Post-Traumatic Stress Disorder (PTSD): Cannabis extracts, specifically lines with better CBD content material material fabric, may additionally moreover assist alleviate signs and symptoms and signs and symptoms of PTSD, collectively with tension and nightmares.

In conclusion, hashish extracts provide a huge variety of benefits and makes use of, each within the medical and entertainment geographical areas. Their recuperation capacity is generally increasing as research delves deeper into the homes of cannabinoids and terpenes. Whether it's miles offering consolation from persistent ache, supplying a steady and effective remedy for epilepsy, or surely enhancing relaxation and creativity, cannabis extracts have cemented their area within the global of nicely-being and interest. However, it's far critical to method their use responsibly and in compliance with community legal guidelines and rules, specifically given the precise results and complexities surrounding those merchandise.

Chapter 11: Types Of Cannabis Extracts

Cannabis extracts are to be had in diverse paperwork, each offering tremendous homes and strategies of intake. These extracts cater to a extensive type of alternatives and dreams, making them a flexible desire for each scientific and leisure clients. In this particular exploration, we can check exquisite varieties of hashish extracts, which includes hash, kief, tinctures, concentrates (shatter, wax, collapse), oils (THC and CBD), edibles, and topicals.

1.   Hash

Hash, quick for hashish, is one of the oldest and most traditional hashish extracts. It is produced with the useful aid of setting apart the trichomes (resin glands) from the hashish plant's plant life. The trichomes are then compressed right into a stable shape, generally a brick or a resinous slab. Hash is to be had in diverse textures and sunglasses, relying on the producing technique and the strain of hashish used. It can be fed on thru

113

smoking, vaporizing, or brought to distinctive hashish products for an extra efficiency enhance.

2.   Kief

Kief is a nice, powdery substance crafted from the trichomes of the cannabis plant. It is often accrued the usage of a grinder with a display that separates the trichomes from the plant fabric. Kief is pretty focused and wealthy in cannabinoids, making it an first-rate addition to joints, bowls, or as a aspect in the manufacturing of different extracts like hash or edibles.

three. Tinctures

Cannabis tinctures are liquid extracts made with the useful resource of dissolving cannabinoids in alcohol or a glycerin base. Tinctures are reachable for specific dosing, as they'll be typically offered in bottles with droppers. They may be fed on sublingually (under the tongue) or introduced to liquids and meals. Tinctures provide speedy onset of outcomes and are a discreet and smoke-free manner to consume cannabis.

4.   Concentrates (Shatter, Wax, Crumble)

Cannabis concentrates are in particular notable extracts recounted for his or her purity and sturdy results. Common sorts of concentrates embody shatter, wax, and collapse, every with its very very personal consistency and texture. These extracts are created via numerous extraction techniques, which consist of butane extraction, CO_2 extraction, or solventless strategies. Concentrates are normally vaporized the use of specialized dab rigs or vaporizers, delivering a sturdy and flavorful enjoy.

Shatter: Shatter is a translucent and glass-like pay hobby that breaks into small quantities. It is known for its immoderate THC content material fabric and purity.

Wax: Cannabis wax has a moderate, wax-like texture and is easy to manipulate. It is favored for its robust outcomes and taste.

Crumble: Crumble is a extra brittle and granulated shape of pay attention. It is prized for its versatility and simplicity of use.

five.   Oils (THC and CBD)

Cannabis oils are bendy extracts which are to be had a liquid form. They may be used for severa features, consisting of oral consumption, vaping, and topical software. These oils can be wealthy in THC, CBD, or a mixture of every, providing a giant form of recovery and leisure results. They are available in fantastic ratios, permitting clients to select out the exceptional oil for his or her precise wishes.

6.   Edibles

Cannabis edibles are a well-known desire for individuals who pick out out a smoke-unfastened and discreet method of consumption. They are available numerous paperwork, in conjunction with gummies, sweets, baked items, and beverages. Edibles are infused with hashish extracts, commonly within the shape of THC or CBD, and provide an prolonged-lasting and doubtlessly more potent revel in in comparison to smoking or vaping. They are stated for his or her not on time onset of results, often taking half of-hour to three hours to kick in.

7.   Topicals

Cannabis-infused topicals are merchandise which might be applied straight away to the pores and pores and pores and skin and are absorbed through the epidermis. These products are generally non-psychoactive, as they do not penetrate the bloodstream. Cannabis topicals, along with creams, creams, balms, and transdermal patches, are regularly used for localized comfort from conditions like pain, inflammation, and pores and skin troubles.

In stop, the world of cannabis extracts is wealthy and numerous, presenting a big range of alternatives for clients to find out. From traditional office work like hash and kief to trendy improvements like concentrates and edibles, each form of extract gives a unique enjoy and advantages. When choosing a cannabis extract, it's miles critical to take into account your choices, preferred outcomes, and intake technique to find out the product that remarkable suits your wishes.

Methods of Extraction

The extraction of cannabinoids and terpenes from the cannabis plant is a essential step in generating numerous cannabis merchandise, inclusive of extracts and concentrates. Different extraction strategies are hired to isolate the ones compounds effectively. In this comprehensive assessment, we will discover not unusual strategies of cannabis extraction, on the facet of solvent-based absolutely extraction (butane, CO_2, ethanol), solventless extraction (dry sift, rosin tech), ice water hash, and the important method of decarboxylation.

1.   Solvent-Based Extraction (Butane, CO_2, Ethanol)

Solvent-based totally definitely sincerely extraction strategies incorporate the usage of a liquid or gasoline to split cannabinoids and terpenes from the hashish plant material. The number one solvents used on this system consist of butane, carbon dioxide (CO2), and ethanol. Each solvent gives specific blessings and produces one in all a kind types of extracts:

Butane Extraction: This approach consists of passing butane thru a cannabis cloth to extract cannabinoids and terpenes, growing merchandise like shatter and wax. Proper purging and safety precautions are essential to do away with residual solvents, as butane is flammable.

CO2 Extraction: Carbon dioxide is substantially seemed as a secure and smooth solvent. It may be utilized in each supercritical and subcritical states to extract a massive sort of cannabinoids and terpenes. CO2 extracts are regularly utilized in vape cartridges and tinctures.

Ethanol Extraction: Ethanol is a flexible solvent for extracting cannabinoids and terpenes. It's commonly taken into consideration greater solid than butane and is frequently used for making tinctures and complete-spectrum cannabis oils. Careful evaporation is needed to take away any residual ethanol.

2.   Solventless Extraction (Dry Sift, Rosin Tech)

Solventless extraction techniques are prized for his or her simplicity and safety, as they do now not comprise the use of probable volatile solvents. Two not unusual solventless extraction techniques are dry sift and rosin tech:

Dry Sift: Dry sift involves routinely putting apart trichomes from the plant material the usage of shows or sieves. This method creates a pleasant, powdery kief, which can be in addition processed into hash or different extracts. It's a conventional and arms-on method.

Rosin Tech: Rosin tech makes use of warmth and stress to extract cannabinoids and terpenes from hashish flower or hash. A rosin press is used to use stress to the cloth, resulting in rosin, a great and terpene-wealthy extract.

three. Ice Water Hash

Ice water hash, additionally referred to as bubble hash, is a solventless extraction approach that uses ice-bloodless water to cut up trichomes from the cannabis plant fabric. The method includes agitating the material with ice water and then the usage of a series of micron bags to clean out the trichomes. The gathered trichomes are then dried and pressed into hashish. Ice water hash is extensively identified for its purity and complete-spectrum individual, because it continues a wide variety of cannabinoids and terpenes.

four. Decarboxylation: Activating the Cannabinoids

Decarboxylation is a crucial step in hashish processing, specially for making edibles, tinctures, and topicals. Cannabis in its uncooked form includes acidic cannabinoids, together with THCA and CBDA, which are non-psychoactive. Decarboxylation involves the software of heat to transform the ones acidic compounds into their lively paperwork, THC and CBD. This technique occurs really while hashish is smoked or vaporized, however at the equal time as making edibles or different non-smokable merchandise, it is crucial to decarboxylate the plant cloth beforehand.

Chapter 12: Equipment And Safety Precautions

Cannabis extraction, whether or now not for non-public use or enterprise production, requires unique machine and adherence to safety measures to make certain a secure and effective device. In this complete dialogue, we're going to discover the important device, protection measures, and the significance of proper air waft and garage even as running with cannabis extracts.

Necessary Equipment

1.   Extraction Vessel: The extraction vessel is the field wherein the cannabis plant material is placed for the extraction approach. Depending at the approach, this vessel may be a closed-loop gadget for solvent-based totally completely extractions or specialised device for solventless techniques.

2.   Solvent Handling Equipment: For solvent-based extractions, specialized device which include closed-loop extraction structures, vacuum ovens, and rotary

evaporators can be essential for coping with and purging solvents nicely.

3.   Filters and Micron Bags: These are utilized in solventless extraction strategies like ice water hash and dry sift to split trichomes from plant material successfully.

4.   Rosin Press: For rosin extraction, a rosin press is wanted to apply warm temperature and stress to the hashish fabric.

5.   Heating and Cooling Equipment: Decarboxylation and other heating strategies require ovens or heating plates, on the same time as cooling system is crucial for keeping safe temperatures at some diploma in the extraction.

6.   PPE (Personal Protective Equipment): Safety equipment which includes gloves, lab coats, and protection glasses defend the extractor from potential exposure to solvents, warm surfaces, or exceptional risks.

Safety Measures

1.   Training and Knowledge: Anyone involved in the extraction method ought to have an extensive understanding of the selected extraction technique, the system used, and safety strategies. Proper schooling is essential to lower risks.

2.   Ventilation: Adequate air float is critical to save you the buildup of in all likelihood risky fumes or vapors. Extraction rooms need to have exhaust structures that successfully do away with solvents or other risky compounds from the air.

three. Fire Safety: Extraction strategies that contain flammable solvents like butane or ethanol require fireplace protection precautions. These may also additionally encompass fireplace suppression structures, explosion-proof gadget, and nicely-ventilated regions to save you the accumulation of flammable vapors.

four. Electrical Safety: Electrical gadget must be nicely grounded and meet safety necessities to reduce the chance of electrical fires or risks.

5. Hazardous Materials Handling: Extractors want to be nicely-versed in handling volatile materials accurately, which include the proper storage, labeling, and disposal of solvents and exclusive chemical compounds.

6. Emergency Response: Facilities want to have emergency reaction plans in vicinity, along with get admission to to hearth extinguishers, eye wash stations, and emergency showers. Personnel should observe in emergency methods.

7. Monitoring and Control: Extraction device need to have automatic safety talents and controls to prevent overheating, overpressurization, or other capacity risks.

Ventilation and Proper Storage

Ventilation and proper storage are important components of protection and maintaining the outstanding of hashish extracts:

1.   Ventilation: Proper air flow is critical to prevent the accumulation of risky fumes and solvents within the extraction environment. Adequate air glide structures must make sure that the extraction vicinity has a ordinary deliver of smooth air and that any risky fumes are efficaciously eliminated. This protects the health of those walking in the facility and minimizes the danger of fireplace or explosion.

2.   Proper Storage: Storing solvents, extraction vessels, and system correctly is critical to keep away from injuries and maintain product extraordinary. Solvents and dangerous materials should be saved in well-ventilated areas, a ways from warmness assets or open flames, and in compliance with close by tips. Cannabis extracts, as quickly as produced, want to be stored in hermetic, moderate-resistant bins to keep their amazing and performance.

In cease, protection is of paramount significance in hashish extraction. Necessary device, safety measures, air waft, and right storage are vital to safeguarding the fitness of these worried within the extraction gadget and making sure the notable of the very last products. Adhering to exceptional practices and recommendations is vital in this evolving enterprise to limit risks and preserve immoderate requirements of protection and product awesome.

Dosage and Consumption of Cannabis

Proper dosage and consumption strategies are critical considerations whilst the usage of hashish, as they immediately impact the outcomes and capability blessings. In this complete talk, we can find out a way to calculate dosage, severa intake techniques (smoking, vaping, ingesting, topical software program program), and the idea of microdosing for a more tailored experience.

Calculating Dosage

Calculating the great dosage of cannabis includes severa factors, including the person's tolerance, experience, and the preferred effects. While there can be nobody-duration-fits-all technique, the subsequent elements can assist decide a suitable region to start:

1.   THC and CBD Content: The awareness of THC and CBD within the product is a important element. High-THC products tend to be more psychoactive, while excessive-CBD merchandise are related to healing consequences with out the "excessive."

2.   Body Weight and Metabolism: A person's frame weight and metabolism will have an effect on how rapid and extraordinarily they enjoy the results of hashish. Generally, people with higher frame weights can also additionally require higher doses.

three. Tolerance: Experienced cannabis customers also can have a better tolerance and require huge doses to achieve the favored consequences.

four. Method of Consumption: Different intake strategies (smoking, vaping, ingesting) result in numerous levels of bioavailability, meaning the body absorbs and strategies cannabinoids in every other manner. For example, ingesting cannabis has a slower onset however longer period of results in evaluation to smoking.

five. Desired Effects: The unique outcomes you're aiming for may want to have an impact on the proper dosage. For instance, pain treatment may additionally moreover require a exclusive dose than rest or creativity.

It's in reality beneficial first of all a low dose and grade by grade increase it over time until you find the proper balance. This technique minimizes the risk of overconsumption and lets in you to gauge how your frame responds to certainly one of a kind dosages.

Consumption Methods

1. Smoking: Smoking cannabis includes respiration in the combusted plant cloth or

concentrates via severa smoking gadgets, which encompass joints, pipes, or bongs. This approach offers rapid onset of effects however may be harsh at the lungs and throat.

2.   Vaping: Vaporizing cannabis entails heating the plant cloth or concentrates to a temperature that releases cannabinoids and terpenes without combustion. Vaping is considered a more wholesome alternative to smoking and offers precise temperature control for a extra customized experience.

3.   Ingesting: Ingesting cannabis includes consuming edibles, pills, or tinctures. The onset of outcomes is slower (usually 30 minutes to 2 hours) however has a tendency to be longer-lasting. Edibles and tablets are available for specific dosing, even as tinctures may be administered sublingually for quicker onset.

4.   Topical Application: Topical merchandise, collectively with creams, balms, and transdermal patches, are implemented

immediately to the pores and pores and skin. These merchandise are non-psychoactive and are in maximum cases used for localized relief from pain, irritation, or pores and skin conditions.

Microdosing

Microdosing includes taking small, sub-healing doses of cannabis to obtain unique, subtle results at the same time as keeping off the acute immoderate related to larger doses. This method is gaining popularity for its capability to enhance attention, creativity, and well-being without impairing daily functioning. Microdosing is specially beneficial for those who need to enjoy the restoration homes of cannabis without experiencing the psychoactive effects.

To microdose effectively, begin with a completely low dose (typically one-tenth of a favored dose) and regularly alter the dosage till you discover the sweet spot in that you experience the popular effects without feeling intoxicated. Microdosing is noticeably individualized, so it may take some experimentation to determine the proper dosage and frequency on your desires.

In give up, expertise the manner to calculate dosage, choosing the right intake approach, and exploring microdosing can significantly beautify your cannabis enjoy. By tailoring your method to your precise desires and selections, you can loosen up the capability benefits of hashish on the identical time as minimizing ability issue results or pain. Always undergo in thoughts to eat responsibly, start with a low dose, and reveal your response to make certain a solid and interesting enjoy.

Chapter 13: Understanding Cannabinoid Ratios

Cannabinoid ratios play a pivotal feature in identifying the effects and capacity blessings of cannabis merchandise. In this complete communicate, we are going to discover the important thing cannabinoids together with THC, CBD, and others, finding the proper balance of these compounds, and the concept of the entourage impact that highlights the importance of the interactions among cannabinoids.

THC, CBD, and Other Cannabinoids

1.   THC (Tetrahydrocannabinol): THC is the number one psychoactive compound in cannabis and is liable for the euphoric "excessive" that many human beings companion with marijuana. It has diverse recovery homes, together with pain relief, anti-nausea consequences, and urge for food stimulation. However, better stages of THC can result in elevated tension or paranoia in a few humans.

2.   CBD (Cannabidiol): CBD is a non-psychoactive cannabinoid with a huge shape of capability recuperation benefits. It is idea for its anti-anxiety, anti-inflammatory, and analgesic homes. CBD also can counteract some of the bad side outcomes of THC, which embody tension and cognitive impairment.

3.   Other Cannabinoids: Besides THC and CBD, there are over 100 special cannabinoids in the hashish plant. Some of the high-quality ones include CBG (cannabigerol), CBN (cannabinol), and THCV (tetrahydrocannabivarin), every with its non-public precise homes and ability benefits.

Finding the Right Balance

The great cannabinoid ratio varies from man or woman to man or woman and is based totally upon on person alternatives and needs. Here are a few issues when finding the proper balance:

1.   Desired Effects: Consider the results you want to acquire. If you searching for rest

and pain consolation without getting excessive, a product with a better CBD to THC ratio can be appropriate. On the alternative hand, if you want to enjoy the euphoric results, a higher THC content material fabric can be preferred.

2. Tolerance: Individual tolerance to cannabinoids can variety notably. People with decrease tolerances may also pick products with a decrease THC content material fabric to avoid pain or overconsumption.

three. Medical Conditions: For particular scientific situations, the right ratio also can additionally range. For instance, some seizure problems respond extremely good to high-CBD, low-THC merchandise, at the same time as conditions like continual ache may additionally moreover additionally benefit from a balanced THC and CBD ratio.

4. Experience Level: Novice customers may need to begin with products that have decrease THC content material cloth fabric to

lessen the functionality for excessive psychoactive outcomes.

5.   Product Type: The form of product you choose can also effect the popular cannabinoid ratio. For instance, edibles often have now not on time onset instances and longer-lasting consequences, making it vital to pick out out a product with the proper stability to your unique desires.

The Entourage Effect

The entourage effect is a idea that highlights the synergistic interplay among numerous cannabinoids and terpenes within the hashish plant. This interaction can decorate the overall healing and psychoactive effects of cannabis. The concept is that the whole plant, with its herbal combination of compounds, gives extra benefits than person cannabinoids in isolation.

For example, some terpenes should have an effect on the results of cannabinoids with the useful aid of modulating their movement at the endocannabinoid device. The presence of a couple of cannabinoids and terpenes can create a unique and custom designed experience for all of us.

To harness the entourage effect, a few customers choose out entire-spectrum or big-spectrum cannabis products, which contain a broader kind of cannabinoids and terpenes in assessment to isolates. These merchandise goal to provide a more properly-rounded and holistic experience.

In give up, knowledge cannabinoid ratios and their consequences is essential for making informed options about cannabis intake. Whether you are seeking out particular recuperation benefits, a particular amusement experience, or are certainly curious about the capacity of cannabinoids, considering the interplay amongst THC, CBD, and special compounds, and exploring the entourage impact, let you discover the right balance to your specific goals. Always start with lower doses and steadily modify as needed to ensure a consistent and fun cannabis enjoy.

Choosing the Right Extract for You

Selecting the proper hashish extract is a custom designed tool that takes below interest your individual opportunities, favored outcomes, scientific wishes, or even the taste and aroma profiles that attraction to you. In this communicate, we can discover the way to make an informed desire primarily based on the ones elements.

Personal Preferences

1. Consumption Method: Your favored approach of intake performs a huge characteristic in choosing the proper cannabis extract. If you select smoking, you will likely select flower or concentrates, on the same time as people who determine on edibles can discover a big variety of infused products.

2. Tolerance and Experience: Your revel in level and tolerance for hashish need to inform your desire. Beginners may moreover

want to begin with merchandise which have a decrease THC content material cloth material to keep away from overwhelming psychoactive consequences.

3. Consistency: Consider whether or not you want a product with regular outcomes and dosing, together with pre-measured edibles, or in case you're comfortable with the variety that can encompass smoking or vaporizing.

Desired Effects

1. Recreational vs. Medicinal: Are you looking for entertainment enjoyment or precise medical advantages? Understanding your primary intention will manual your desire of extract. High-THC extracts are much more likely to supply euphoric effects, while excessive-CBD extracts are regularly used for healing functions.

2. Specific Effects: Think approximately the consequences you preference. Do you need to loosen up, enhance creativity, or

alleviate unique signs and symptoms like ache or anxiety? Different extracts can deliver wonderful results, so pick out one which aligns collectively together with your desires.

three. Duration of Effects: Consider how long you need the results to final. Smoking or vaping can also additionally offer quicker onset and shorter duration, on the same time as edibles offer a slower onset and longer-lasting consequences.

Medical Needs

1. Condition and Symptoms: If you've got were given were given particular scientific situations or symptoms and signs and symptoms you need to cope with, studies which cannabinoids and terpenes are effective to your desires. For example, CBD-wealthy extracts are often used for epilepsy and anxiety, at the same time as high-THC merchandise can be appropriate for ache control.

2.   Dosage Control: If you require particular dosing, don't forget products that provide smooth and correct dosing options, which incorporates tinctures or pills.

three. Consult with a Healthcare Professional: If you've got got were given crucial medical issues or are the usage of cannabis to update or supplement modern remedies, it is suggested to are looking for advice from a healthcare expert who has revel in with hashish remedy.

Flavor and Aroma Profiles

1.   Terpenes: Terpenes are chargeable for the tremendous flavors and aromas of hashish extracts. If you apprehend unique flavors or aromas, studies the terpene profiles of diverse traces to discover extracts that in form your alternatives.

2.   Strain Specificity: Some humans pick out to paste to particular cannabis strains recognized for his or her unique taste and

aroma profiles. This can upload a layer of customization for your hashish experience.

three. Experimentation: If you are open to exploring new taste and aroma profiles, you could check with top notch extracts to find out new and thrilling terpene mixtures.

In end, selecting the proper cannabis extract is a deeply personal selection that relies upon on your options, desires, scientific dreams, or even sensory tales. By carefully considering the elements referred to above, you can select out the extract that aligns together with your individual tastes and goals. Remember to start with decrease doses, especially in case you're new to hashish or attempting a new product, to ensure a steady and a laugh revel in.

Chapter 14: Purchasing And Storing Cannabis Extracts

Once you have got decided at the right hashish extract on your dreams, it is crucial to recognize a way to buy it, shop it well, and understand its shelf life and safety. In this comprehensive communicate, we can find out the options for acquiring cannabis extracts, right garage techniques, and a way to maintain the fantastic of your products through the years.

Dispensaries and Online Options

1.   Dispensaries: Dispensaries   are regulated stores in which you should purchase hashish products, along with extracts. They provide a exquisite fashion of alternatives, and informed personnel will let you make informed alternatives primarily based in your alternatives and goals. When travelling a dispensary, ensure you have were given a valid ID and, in a few times, a scientific marijuana card if required via your jurisdiction.

2.   Online Retailers: Many areas permit the web purchase of cannabis extracts. Buying online gives comfort and a broader choice, and you could regularly discover unique product descriptions and evaluations. Ensure

you're buying from a good, licensed supply, and be aware of the criminal guidelines concerning on line hashish purchases in your region.

Proper Storage Techniques

1.   Temperature and Humidity: Cannabis extracts need to be stored in a cool, dry location. Excessive warmth or humidity can degrade the exceptional of the product and motive mildew or mould to increase. Room temperature (round 70°F or 21°C) is normally perfect.

2.   Airtight Containers: To prevent oxidation and preserve freshness, use hermetic packing containers, collectively with glass jars or silicone containers, to keep your extracts. These packing containers help keep the product's flavor, aroma, and efficiency.

3.   Light Protection: Cannabis extracts are sensitive to moderate, that could degrade cannabinoids and terpenes through the years. Keep your products in opaque bins, or keep

them in a dark location to shield them from mild exposure.

four. Avoid Oxygen Exposure: Oxygen can bring about the degradation of cannabinoids. Vacuum-sealed packaging or using nitrogen gasoline to displace oxygen may be effective techniques for upkeep.

5. Refrigeration or Freezing: Some extracts, mainly perishable edibles, can advantage from refrigeration or freezing to boom shelf lifestyles. However, this isn't encouraged for all merchandise, as freezing can cause modifications in texture and consistency.

Shelf Life and Preservation

1. Expiration Dates: Check the product labels for expiration dates or "great through" dates. These dates are furnished via manufacturers to ensure product super and safety.

2. Product Rotation: If you have got have been given a couple of hashish extracts, take

into account of product rotation. Consume older products in advance than extra moderen ones to make sure you enjoy the extracts at their pinnacle freshness.

three. Avoid Contamination: Prevent infection thru the usage of smooth utensils and fending off touching the product together collectively along with your arms. Residue from your hands can introduce impurities and degrade the product over the years.

4. Testing: Some jurisdictions require hashish products to go through checking out for purity and efficiency. Ensure that the products you buy have been examined with the aid of way of the usage of respectable labs to assure safety and first-rate.

5. Dosage Awareness: Be aware of the advocated dosage and begin with decrease doses, especially whilst attempting new merchandise. This can help prevent overconsumption and functionality element results.

In conclusion, buying and storing cannabis extracts involves making knowledgeable alternatives and taking precautions to maintain product splendid and safety. Whether you pick out a close-by dispensary or on-line store, make sure that you are shopping from a criminal, licensed source. Proper storage techniques, along facet temperature manipulate, airtight containers, and safety from mild and oxygen, are vital to maintain the extraordinary of your extracts. By following those suggestions, you may experience your cannabis extracts to the fullest and experience their intended consequences at the identical time as minimizing functionality degradation over time.

Potential Risks and Side Effects of Cannabis Extracts

Cannabis extracts provide quite a number of advantages, however like severa substance, similarly they encompass capability risks and thing effects. In this whole communicate, we are going to find out the fast-term and lengthy-time period risks related to cannabis extracts, strategies to mitigate capability aspect consequences, and a manner to understand allergies.

Short-Term Risks and Side Effects

1.   Impaired Coordination: Short-term cannabis use can impair coordination, main to reduced motor capabilities and an extended threat of injuries.

2.   Cognitive Impairment: Cannabis can short have an effect on cognitive feature, fundamental to reminiscence and interest troubles, which can be in particular tough for duties requiring cognizance.

3.   Anxiety and Paranoia: High-THC merchandise, specially in immoderate doses or for green customers, can cause tension, paranoia, and improved coronary heart fee.

4.   Dry Mouth and Red Eyes: Commonly called "cottonmouth," hashish use frequently

results in a dry mouth, together with pink, bloodshot eyes.

5.   Increased Appetite: Cannabis can stimulate urge for meals, often referred to as "the munchies," which also can cause overeating.

6.   Psychoactive Effects: Depending on the THC content, cannabis extracts can set off psychoactive results along side euphoria, altered belief of time, and sensory enhancements.

Long-Term Risks

1.   Addiction: While not all and sundry who makes use of cannabis turns into addicted, lengthy-term, heavy use can bring about dependency, characterised via withdrawal signs and signs and symptoms while looking for to quit.

2.   Mental Health: Some people may be at an progressed threat of highbrow fitness problems, which incorporates despair, tension, and psychosis, specially within the

occasion that they have a circle of relatives statistics of intellectual fitness issues.

3. Respiratory Issues: Smoking hashish can purpose respiratory troubles, just like tobacco, collectively with bronchitis and lung troubles.

4. Reduced Lung Function: Long-time period use of immoderate-THC merchandise can motive reduced lung function.

Mitigating Potential Side Effects

1. Dosage Control: Start with low doses, specifically if you're a novice or attempting a modern-day product. Gradually boom the dosage as had to mitigate functionality aspect consequences.

2. Choose the Right Strain: Different cannabis lines have diverse results. If you're liable to anxiety or paranoia, don't forget lines with a balanced THC to CBD ratio or select high-CBD extracts.

3.   Controlled Environment: Use cannabis in a steady and acquainted surroundings, in that you feel cushty and strong.

four.   Hydration: To counteract dry mouth, live properly-hydrated at the equal time as the usage of hashish.

five.   Avoid Overconsumption: Pace your consumption to avoid overeating, specifically in case you're susceptible to the munchies.

6.   Limit Use: Practice moderation and keep away from extended-term, heavy use to decrease the chance of dependency and particular prolonged-term fitness problems.

Recognizing Allergic Reactions

Cannabis allergies are uncommon but can arise. Symptoms of allergies may additionally consist of:

Skin rashes or hives

Itchy or watery eyes

Congestion or sneezing

Nausea or vomiting

Swelling of the face, lips, or tongue

Difficulty respiratory

If you enjoy any of those signs and signs and signs and symptoms after consuming hashish extracts, prevent use right now and are searching out scientific hobby if the signs and symptoms persist or get worse. It's additionally important to tell healthcare companies about your cannabis use, as cannabis hypersensitive reactions can be just like one of a kind hypersensitive reactions and can require particular treatments.

Chapter 15: Legal Considerations And Regulations

Cannabis laws and tips range widely spherical the sector, making it vital to understand the criminal panorama, together with federal and kingdom legal guidelines, variations amongst clinical and amusement hashish, and troubles for visiting with hashish extracts.

Federal and State Laws

1.   Federal Laws: In the USA, hashish remains illegal beneath federal law as a Schedule I managed substance, which makes its ownership, sale, and use a federal offense. Federal enforcement of hashish criminal tips can variety primarily based completely totally on political and law enforcement priorities.

2.   State Laws: Cannabis felony recommendations are in the critical dominated on the kingdom diploma. As of my last information update in September 2021, a developing widespread type of U.S. States have legalized cannabis for every scientific and leisure use. Each u . S . Has its very very

own set of regulations, which incorporates age limits, possession limits, and licensing requirements for companies.

3.   International Laws: Cannabis felony suggestions furthermore variety substantially internationally, with a few international locations genuinely legalizing entertainment and scientific hashish, at the identical time as others holds strict prohibition.

Medical vs. Recreational Cannabis

1.   Medical Cannabis: Many jurisdictions have legalized scientific hashish, permitting sufferers with qualifying situations to obtain cannabis products, together with extracts, with a scientific medical doctor's advice or prescription. Medical cannabis programs normally have stricter rules governing affected individual eligibility and the forms of products available.

2.   Recreational Cannabis: Recreational hashish is criminal in severa states and worldwide places, permitting adults of a

excessive exceptional age to buy and use cannabis products for non-clinical capabilities. These policies also can allow severa varieties of hashish extracts, counting on community legal guidelines.

three. Age Restrictions: Both medical and leisure hashish packages regularly have age regulations in place, typically requiring human beings to be as a minimum 18 or 21 years antique to buy and very own cannabis products.

Traveling with Cannabis Extracts

1. Domestic Travel: When visiting interior a country wherein cannabis is legal, it is crucial to recognize neighborhood laws and regulations regarding the transportation of hashish extracts. In the us, as an instance, it's miles normally unlawful to move hashish all through kingdom traces, even among states with jail hashish.

2. International Travel: Traveling across the world with cannabis extracts may be

complex and unstable. Many countries have strict drug laws, or perhaps the ownership of a small quantity of hashish can bring about immoderate prison effects. Research an appropriate prison hints of the holiday spot the united states and the potential effects in advance than attempting to tour with cannabis.

3.   Air Travel: The Transportation Security Administration (TSA) in the United States has stated that its primary hobby is on protection and no longer the invention of illegal tablets. However, if hashish is found to your possession within the course of an airport safety test, TSA may additionally refer the matter to law enforcement, specially if it is prohibited beneath neighborhood or federal regulation.

four. Compliance with Local Laws: Whether journeying regionally or across the world, constantly ensure compliance with network legal guidelines. This consists of analyzing the legal guidelines of your departure and arrival places, and respecting the rules and regulations of the airport or airline.

Please be conscious that cannabis crook recommendations and regulations are normally evolving, and changes can upward push up after my closing knowledge replace in September 2021. Therefore, it's miles vital to live updated on the cutting-edge prison repute of cannabis in your location and any locations you want to visit, in addition to to comply with all applicable prison recommendations and recommendations to avoid criminal troubles.

CHAPER 12: Interactions and Contraindications of Cannabis Extracts

Using cannabis extracts should be executed with caution, as they're able to engage with unique materials and characteristic precise contraindications, specifically almost approximately drug interactions, combining with alcohol, and special concerns for high quality medical situations. In this complete communicate, we are going to find out these important elements.

Drug Interactions

Cannabis extracts could have interplay with diverse prescription and over-the-counter drugs, in all likelihood foremost to destructive results. It's vital to speak approximately with a healthcare professional if you're taking one-of-a-kind drugs and thinking about using hashish extracts. Here are some functionality interactions to be privy to:

1.   Central Nervous System Depressants: Cannabis can decorate the consequences of critical anxious tool depressants, consisting of sedatives, hypnotics, and sure pain medicines. Combining these substances can result in elevated drowsiness, dizziness, and impaired coordination.

2.   Blood Thinners: Cannabis extracts, particularly high-THC merchandise, may additionally boom the threat of bleeding while used alongside element blood thinners

like warfarin or certain antiplatelet medicinal drugs.

three. Antipsychotic Medications: Combining hashish with antipsychotic medicinal drugs may additionally moreover have complicated effects. In some instances, hashish may also moreover lessen the effectiveness of antipsychotic capsules.

four. Certain Antidepressants: Cannabis can also interact with selective serotonin reuptake inhibitors (SSRIs) and monoamine oxidase inhibitors (MAOIs), possibly inflicting unfavourable reactions, together with serotonin syndrome.

5. Opioid Medications: Using hashish alongside opioid medicinal capsules can increase the sedative effects and can result in extra drowsiness, respiration melancholy, and a higher threat of overdose.

6. Antiepileptic Drugs: The interplay amongst cannabis and antiepileptic capsules may be complex. While a few sufferers use

CBD-wealthy cannabis extracts to control seizures, THC can lessen the effectiveness of a few antiepileptic medicines.

Combining with Alcohol

Combining hashish extracts with alcohol can motive extra positive effects and stepped forward impairment. Both materials have depressant homes and may impair motor competencies, cognitive feature, and judgment. The aggregate can bring about:

1.   Increased Intoxication: When alcohol and hashish are used collectively, intoxication also can moreover arise greater rapid and really, essential to terrible choice-making and a better risk of accidents.

2.   Impaired Coordination: The mixture can result in decreased coordination, affecting sports activities together with using or operating heavy equipment.

three. Cognitive Impairment: Both alcohol and cannabis can motive cognitive impairment, along side memory issues and attention problems, which is probably exacerbated while used collectively.

4.	Increased Risk: Combining alcohol and hashish can result in various health dangers, such as an extended probability of addiction, blackouts, and substance abuse troubles.

Special Considerations for Certain Medical Conditions

1.	Heart Conditions: Cannabis can in short growth coronary heart fee and blood strain. If you have coronary coronary heart conditions or a information of coronary coronary heart infection, talk over with a healthcare professional before the usage of hashish extracts, mainly those excessive in THC.

2.	Psychiatric Disorders: Individuals with a information of psychiatric issues, collectively with schizophrenia or bipolar disease, can be greater vulnerable to the capacity psychoactive effects of hashish, that can exacerbate signs and signs and signs and symptoms. A healthcare professional's steerage is critical inside the ones times.

3. Respiratory Conditions: Smoking cannabis extracts can worsen the lungs and exacerbate breathing situations, which include allergies or continual obstructive pulmonary illness (COPD). Alternative consumption techniques like vaping or edibles may be very last for human beings with breathing troubles.

four. Pregnancy and Breastfeeding: The use of hashish extracts in the course of being pregnant and breastfeeding is discouraged because of potential damage to the developing fetus or toddler. Consult with a healthcare professional for steering in case you're pregnant or breastfeeding.

five. Pediatric Patients: Cannabis use in kids and youngsters need to handiest be taken into consideration below the guidance of a healthcare professional and while different remedies have established ineffective.

In conclusion, interactions and contraindications of hashish extracts should be taken significantly. It's important to speak about with a healthcare expert, in particular if you have pre-gift medical conditions or are taking other medicinal drugs. Being aware about capacity drug interactions, fending off combining cannabis with alcohol, and considering the particular needs and sensitivities of great clinical situations can assist ensure a secure and responsible use of cannabis extracts.

Chapter 16: Tips For Positive Cannabis Extract Experience

An exceptional revel in with hashish extracts requires cautious attention of your surroundings, accountable use, and hobby of social and crook elements. In this communicate; we are able to discover crucial recommendations to make certain a stable and thrilling cannabis extract experience.

Setting and Setting

1.   Choose the Right Environment: Select a comfortable and acquainted environment, preferably loose from distractions or stressors. Your setting performs a vital feature within the way you experience cannabis, so create a location in that you enjoy comfortable and regular.

2.   Mindset Matters: Ensure that you're in a tremendous mind-set while the usage of hashish. If you are feeling disturbing, forced, or disillusioned, it's miles absolutely beneficial to wait till you are in a better frame of mind, as hashish can increase your feelings.

3.   Prepare Necessities: Have the whole lot you need internal achieve, along with water, snacks, entertainment, and any system required for your selected intake technique. This minimizes the need to transport round and lets in you stay cushty.

Responsible Use

1.   Start with a Low Dose: Especially in case you're new to cannabis or trying a today's product, start with a low dose. You can generally eat extra if needed, but it is difficult to contrary the results of overconsumption.

2.   Time Your Consumption: Consider the timing of your hashish use. If you have got responsibilities or duties, make sure your consumption may not intervene with them, and which you have sufficient time for the experience.

3.   Stay Hydrated: Cannabis can motive dry mouth, so have water available to stay hydrated.

4.   Know Your Tolerance: If you're an expert individual, be aware of your tolerance and adjust your dosage as a end result.

5.   Don't Drive Under the Influence: Never electricity or function heavy system whilst below the have an effect on of hashish extracts, as it impairs motor abilties and judgment.

6.   Avoid Combining Substances: Avoid mixing cannabis extracts with alcohol or different substances, as it is able to bring about unpredictable results and heightened impairment.

Social and Legal Considerations

1.   Respect Local Laws: Stay informed about the crook hints and guidelines related to hashish for your location. Compliance with nearby criminal tips is critical to avoid jail troubles.

2.   Social Considerations: If you're the usage of cannabis with others, make certain that they may be comfortable with it and

which you're in a consistent, supportive social placing.

three. Confidentiality: Keep your hashish use different if wanted, especially in conditions wherein it may have professional or criminal implications.

4. Monitor and Adjust: Pay interest to how you feel, and be prepared to modify your surroundings or consumption in case you enjoy ache or unexpected consequences.

five. Seek Medical Help if Needed: In the occasion of intense horrible results, which encompass tension or paranoia, or in case you suspect an overdose, are looking for clinical hobby right away.

6. Responsible Storage: If you've got got children or pets, make sure that your cannabis extracts are securely saved and out in their reap.

In conclusion, a wonderful cannabis extract revel in is based totally upon on your placing, accountable use, and data of social and crook problems. By growing a cushty environment, the use of hashish responsibly, and respecting nearby legal hints and social dynamics, you could revel in the functionality benefits of cannabis extracts while minimizing potential dangers. Always prioritize protection and well-being when the usage of hashish extracts.

Chapter 17: Frequently Asked Questions

Cannabis extracts can be complicated, and those regularly have questions about severa components in their use. In this phase, we're going to address some common problems and inquiries associated with cannabis extracts.

1.   What are hashish extracts, and the way are they awesome from ordinary cannabis?

Cannabis extracts are focused styles of hashish, wherein the plant's cannabinoids and terpenes are extracted to create merchandise like oils, concentrates, tinctures, and edibles. These extracts usually have better efficiency and a awesome chemical profile in evaluation to standard cannabis flower.

2.   What are the capability medical benefits of hashish extracts?

Cannabis extracts have been used to manipulate numerous medical conditions, together with persistent pain, epilepsy, tension, and nausea. CBD-rich extracts are regularly looked for their ability restoration blessings, at the same time as THC-rich extracts may be used for ache comfort and relaxation.

three. Are cannabis extracts jail?

The crook popularity of cannabis extracts varies by means of area. In some locations, they are jail for each clinical and leisure use, even as in others, they'll be prohibited or constrained. It's important to understand and study close by prison tips and regulations.

Chapter 18: An Overview Of Cbd Oil

CBD oil, furthermore referred to as cannabidiol oil, has grown in popularity as a flexible properly being product, taking photographs the eye of those searching for herbal solutions to numerous fitness problems. CBD is a non-psychoactive molecule crafted from the hashish plant, which means that it does not provide the "high" that THC does. As the jail surroundings surrounding cannabis has superior, CBD has obtained momentum for its capability scientific homes, ensuing in a surge in its reputation for the duration of the area.

CBD oil is generated with the aid of the usage of and big from hemp, a form of hashish with a low THC interest. This extraction approach involves retaining apart CBD from wonderful cannabinoids and plant components to create a focused form of it. The resulting oil may be fed on sublingually, topically, or on the equal time as a meal. The beauty of CBD oil arises from its purported capability to remedy a massive kind of illnesses, from anxiety and chronic pain to sleep issues, with out the destructive outcomes related to many drug treatments.

CBD's Origins And History

While CBD's modern prominence indicates a smooth discovery, it's been spherical for millennia. Cannabis has been implemented medicinally because of the fact that historic civilizations to deal with a massive range of fitness troubles. CBD, however, wasn't separated as a outstanding detail until the mid-20th century.

In 1940, Dr. Roger Adams and his colleagues isolated CBD from the hashish plant. Dr. Raphael Mechoulam, dubbed the "Father of Cannabis Research," did now not discover the CBD shape till the Nineteen Sixties. Dr. Mechoulam's landmark discovery paved the way for in addition studies into the compound's potential medical homes.

CBD has grown in prominence because of its anticonvulsant homes in the course of the years. The case of Charlotte Figi, a piece little one with intense epilepsy, sparked large hobby within the early twenty-first century. Her story, which have become appreciably posted, determined out CBD's potential to reduce the frequency and severity of seizures, inspiring in addition research and public interest.

The passage of the 2018 Farm Bill in the United States marked a turning factor for CBD. This act legalized hemp manufacturing, distinguishing it from marijuana and putting off criminal barriers to CBD's big dissemination. As a end result, CBD merchandise, in particular oils, have grow to be greater with out issues available, helping the enterprise's rapid boom.

CBD includes cannabinoids, which can be chemical materials.

CBD is a chemical compound that belongs to the cannabis beauty. These compounds have interaction with the endocannabinoid tool (ECS) of the human body, influencing numerous physiological approaches. While the cannabis plant contains over a hundred cannabinoids, CBD and THC are the most famous and investigated.

Despite having the equal chemical approach (21 carbon atoms, 30 hydrogen atoms, and oxygen atoms), the atomic configurations of CBD and THC range, ensuing in remarkable results. CBD, in comparison to THC, does no longer bind strongly to the critical worried gadget cannabinoid receptors CB1 and CB2, and is the reason why it is non-psychoactive.

Cannabinoids and the ECS have interaction in a complex style, influencing neurotransmitter launch, immunological responses, and the stability of many physiological features. CBD's capability to have interaction with the ECS without generating a "high" makes it a promising recovery method.

An Introduction To The Endocannabinoid System

The endocannabinoid device (ECS) is critical for body homeostasis. Endocannabinoids, receptors, and enzymes include this tool, which emerge as identified inside the late Nineteen Eighties. Endocannabinoids bind to receptors in the body to alter a number of sports activities, consisting of temper, sleep, urge for food, and immune response.

CB1 receptors, which might be predominantly determined in the significant disturbing tool, and CB2 receptors, which can be by means of way of and massive located within the peripheral concerned machine and immune cells, are the 2 types of receptors gift inside the ECS. Endocannabinoids bind to those receptors like keys to locks, evoking physiological responses that assist the frame keep equilibrium.

CBD affects receptor activity, interacting with the ECS. While it does not immediately bind to CB1 and CB2 receptors, it does modify their interest, enhancing the body's herbal endocannabinoid manufacturing. This indirect link contributes to CBD's healing blessings, giving a holistic approach for supporting the ECS in retaining stability.

Classifications Of CBD Oil

CBD oil is to be had in numerous forms, every catering to a particular set of opportunities and dreams. The 3 vital sorts are entire-spectrum, sizeable-spectrum, and CBD isolate.

1. Full-spectrum CBD Oil includes a numerous shape of cannabinoids, terpenes, and one-of-a-kind medicinal additives derived from the cannabis plant. There are trace amounts of THC in this, but no longer enough to be psychoactive. The "entourage impact," a synergistic interplay amongst those compounds, is expected to decorate CBD's clinical benefits. Whole-spectrum oils are recommended for individuals who want to revel in the whole spectrum of cannabis compounds and their numerous combinations.

2. Broad-Spectrum CBD Oil: Broad-spectrum CBD oil, like complete-spectrum CBD oil, has pretty a variety of cannabinoids and terpenes however does no longer include THC. This approach is right for folks that want to revel in the entourage effect but are not in a position to perform that because of crook restrictions or personal possibilities. Broad-spectrum CBD gives an entire method to remedy even as maintaining off THC intoxication.

three. CBD Isolate is the purest shape of CBD, which consist of 99% pure CBD with out a extraordinary cannabinoids or plant compounds. Because the isolation system gets rid of all traces of THC and other additives, it is an exquisite choice for those who desire the blessings of CBD with out the danger of THC exposure. CBD isolation is commonly desired by using way of oldsters which might be sensitive to distinctive cannabinoids or who are required to post to drug checking out.

Finally, the transition of CBD oil from historical medicinal use to fashionable-day nicely being darling indicates the evolving hashish splendor weather. Because of its wealthy statistics, complicated chemical interactions, and severa product offerings, CBD oil maintains to make its claim in the arena of herbal health solutions, bringing a international of possibilities for absolutely everyone attempting to find a holistic approach to well-being.

Methods of CBD Extraction

CBD (cannabidiol) oil has acquired in popularity due to its capability fitness advantages, and the extraction approach is important in figuring out the exceptional and purity of the finished product. There are various techniques for extracting CBD from the cannabis plant, each with its non-public set of benefits and disadvantages.

The CO_2 extraction method is a common extraction technique. This approach employs carbon dioxide in a supercritical kingdom, which has the homes of each a liquid and a gasoline. In this diploma, CO_2 acts as a solvent, disposing of suitable compounds from the cannabis plant, which consist of cannabinoids like CBD. CO_2 extraction produces tremendous CBD oil without using poisonous solvents, resulting in a natural and sturdy product.

Ethanol extraction is each extraordinary technique that employs ethanol (ethyl alcohol) as a solvent. This manner is each cheap and effective, however, it may do away with no longer best CBD however additionally certainly one of a type additives like chlorophyll, ensuing in lots less herbal output. Impurities inside the recovered oil after ethanol extraction also can want further processing.

As hydrocarbon extraction techniques, butane and propane extraction are also used. Although residual solvents can also stay in the end product if no longer completely purged, the ones solvents efficaciously extract cannabinoids from plant material. This will increase worries about safety due to the fact those solvents are flammable and likely volatile if consumed.

Lipid extraction is a miles less common approach of hashish absorption and extraction that consists of the use of fats or lipids. This technique is typically used to create infused oils, however, it can now not be as a hit at extracting huge levels of CBD as particular strategies.

A variety of things have an effect on the extraction method employed, which includes the supposed give up product, financial concerns, and safety troubles. Manufacturers ought to examine proper manufacturing techniques and do entire trying out to guarantee that the completed CBD oil is freed from impurities and fulfills exceptional requirements.

Understanding The THC And CBD Relationship

THC (tetrahydrocannabinol) and CBD (cannabidiol) are of the hashish plant's maximum well-known cannabinoids. Both have recovery homes, however their psychotropic effects are not the same. Customers searching out particular medicinal advantages without the "high" related to THC want to recognize the CBD-to-THC ratios in a certain product.

CBD and THC each engage with the endocannabinoid tool (ECS) of the human frame but in exceptional strategies. CBD is non-psychotropic and is taken into consideration to mitigate THC's consequences. When CBD and THC are combined, they might cause what is referred to as the "entourage impact," in which the mixed cannabinoids enhance the medicinal outcomes of every one-of-a-kind.

The CBD-to-THC ratio of various lines of cannabis and hemp vegetation varies, and this ratio is a huge trouble in determining a product's consequences. Products with a immoderate CBD-to-THC ratio are much more likely to deliver medicinal benefits whilst displaying no detectable psychoactive effect. Individuals who want to keep away from the intoxicating consequences of THC and get treatment for illnesses like tension, ache, and irritation typically pick these merchandise.

Higher THC-content cloth material merchandise, on the other hand, can be counseled for times wherein euphoric effects are sought, which includes controlling some varieties of pain or boosting urge for meals in chemotherapy sufferers.

Both medical examiners and clients need to apprehend the ones ratios to make informed judgments regarding the acceptability of a product for a sure reason.

THC interest recommendations in CBD merchandise variety through place, so clients need to be aware about neighborhood criminal pointers and pick out out gadgets that meet their tastes further to criminal dreams.

CBD Oil Health Advantages

CBD oil has gotten quite a few hobby because of its possible health benefits for a lot of ailments. CBD appears to interact with the endocannabinoid device, which regulates quite a few physiological capabilities which includes temper, sleep, hunger, and immunological feature.

One of the most famous CBD advantages is its functionality to alleviate continual pain. CBD has been established in studies to alleviate pain with the aid of influencing endocannabinoid receptor feature, reducing infection, and interacting with neurotransmitters. As a end end result, CBD is a possible treatment choice for people stricken by illnesses like arthritis, more than one sclerosis, or chronic ache syndromes.

CBD has moreover confirmed promise in lowering anxiety and despair symptoms and signs. It binds to serotonin receptors inside the thoughts, converting temper and provoking rest.

Some users suggest that it permits them manage social anxiety, positioned up-annoying pressure ailment (PTSD), and generalized tension disease (GAD).

CBD may additionally have neuroprotective developments, implying a role inside the treatment of neurological ailments. Although studies is ongoing, there is proof that CBD can be useful in ailments at the side of epilepsy, Alzheimer's disorder, and Parkinson's sickness.

CBD's anti-inflammatory traits make it a possible opportunity for pores and skin care products, thinking about it may aid within the remedy of troubles which includes zits and eczema. Its antioxidant capabilities assist to maintain pores and pores and skin fitness thru neutralizing unfastened radicals that reason harm and untimely developing older.